INTERVENTIONAL CARDIOLOGY CLINICS

www.interventional.theclinics.com

Editor-in-Chief

MATTHEW J. PRICE

Congenital Heart Disease Intervention

January 2019 • Volume 8 • Number 1

Editor

DANIEL S. LEVI

ELSEVIER

1600 John F. Kennedy Boulevard • Suite 1800 • Philadelphia, Pennsylvania, 19103-2899

http://www.theclinics.com

INTERVENTIONAL CARDIOLOGY CLINICS Volume 8, Number 1
January 2019 ISSN 2211-7458, ISBN-13: 978-0-323-65499-9

Editor: Lauren Boyle
Developmental Editor: Donald Mumford

Interventional Cardiology Clinics (ISSN 2211-7458) is published quarterly by Elsevier Inc., 360 Park Avenue South, New York, NY 10010-1710. Months of issue are January, April, July, and October. Subscription prices are USD 203 per year for US individuals, USD 474 for US institutions, USD 100 per year for US students, USD 204 per year for Canadian individuals, USD 565 for Canadian institutions, USD 150 per year for Canadian students, USD 296 per year for international individuals, USD 565 for international institutions, and USD 150 per year for international students. To receive student/resident rate, orders must be accompanied by name of affiliated institution, date of term, and the *signature* of program/residency coordinator on institution letterhead. Orders will be billed at individual rate until proof of status is received. Foreign air speed delivery is included in all *Clinics* subscription prices. All prices are subject to change without notice. **POSTMASTER:** Send address changes to *Interventional Cardiology Clinics*, Elsevier Health Sciences Division, Subscription Customer Service, 3251 Riverport Lane, Maryland Heights, MO 63043. **Customer Service: Telephone: 1-800-654-2452** (U.S. and Canada); **1-314-447-8871** (outside U.S. and Canada). **Fax: 1-314-447-8029. E-mail: journalscustomerservice-usa@elsevier.com (for print support); journalsonlinesupport-usa@elsevier.com (for online support).**

Reprints. For copies of 100 or more of articles in this publication, please contact the Commercial Reprints Department, Elsevier Inc., 360 Park Avenue South, New York, NY 10010-1710. Tel.: 212-633-3874; Fax: 212-633-3820; E-mail: reprints@elsevier.com.

CONTRIBUTORS

EDITOR-IN-CHIEF

MATTHEW J. PRICE, MD
Director, Cardiac Catheterization Laboratory,
Division of Cardiovascular Diseases, Scripps
Clinic, Assistant Professor, Scripps
Translational Science Institute, La Jolla,
California

EDITOR

DANIEL S. LEVI, MD
Professor of Pediatrics, UCLA Pediatrics,
Director of Pediatric and Adult Congenital
Catheterization Laboratory at UCLA, Division
of Pediatric Cardiology, UCLA
Mattel Children's Hospital, Los Angeles,
California

AUTHORS

JAMIL ABOULHOSN, MD
Department of Medicine, Division of
Cardiology, Ahmanson/UCLA Adult
Congenital Heart Disease Center, Ronald
Reagan UCLA Medical Center, Los Angeles,
California

HITESH AGRAWAL, MD
Assistant Professor of Pediatrics,
Pediatric Interventional Cardiology,
The University of Tennessee, LeBonheur
Children's Hospital, Memphis,
Tennessee

SAROSH P. BATLIVALA, MD, MSCI
Associate Professor of Pediatrics,
The Heart Institute, Cincinnati Children's
Hospital Medical Center, Cincinnati,
Ohio

BRYAN H. GOLDSTEIN, MD
Associate Professor of Pediatrics,
Associate Director, Cardiac Catheterization
and Intervention, The Heart
Institute, Cincinnati Children's
Hospital Medical Center, Cincinnati,
Ohio

DANIEL S. LEVI, MD
Professor of Pediatrics, UCLA Pediatrics,
Director of Pediatric and Adult Congenital
Catheterization Laboratory at UCLA, Division
of Pediatric Cardiology, UCLA
Mattel Children's Hospital, Los Angeles,
California

GARETH J. MORGAN, MB, BaO, BCh
Department of Pediatric Cardiology,
Children's Hospital of Colorado, University of
Colorado School of Medicine, Aurora,
Colorado

BRIAN H. MORRAY, MD
Assistant Professor, Pediatrics,
Division of Pediatric Cardiology, Seattle
Children's Hospital, University of
Washington School of Medicine, Seattle,
Washington

ALAN W. NUGENT, MBBS, FRACP
Division of Cardiology, Professor, Department
of Pediatrics, Northwestern University
Feinberg School of Medicine, Ann & Robert H.
Lurie Children's Hospital of Chicago, Chicago,
Illinois

MICHAEL L. O'BYRNE, MD, MSCE
Assistant Professor of Pediatrics, Division of
Cardiology and Center for Pediatric Clinical
Effectiveness, The Children's Hospital of
Philadelphia, Department of Pediatrics,
Cardiovascular Outcomes, Quality, and
Evaluate Research Center, Leonard Davis
Institute, Perelman School of Medicine,
University of Pennsylvania, Philadelphia,
Pennsylvania

SHYAM SATHANANDAM, MD, FSCAI
Medical Director of the Invasive Cardiac
Imaging and Interventional Catheterization
Laboratory, Department of Pediatric
Interventional Cardiology, The University of
Tennessee, LeBonheur Children's Hospital,
Memphis, Tennessee

SANJAY SINHA, MD
Assistant Professor, Department of Pediatrics,
Division of Cardiology, UCLA Mattel
Children's Hospital, Los Angeles, California

SUSHITHA SURENDAN, MD
Assistant Professor of Pediatrics and Pediatric
Cardiology, Department of Pediatric
Interventional Cardiology, The University of
Tennessee, LeBonheur Children's Hospital,
Memphis, Tennessee

**SURENDRANATH R. VEERAM REDDY, MD,
FSCAI**
Division of Cardiology, Associate Professor,
Department of Pediatrics, The University of
Texas Southwestern Medical Center,
Children's Health System of Texas, Children's
Medical Center, Dallas, Texas

BENJAMIN RUSH WALLER III, MD
Professor of Pediatrics, Pediatric
Interventional Cardiology, The University of
Tennessee, LeBonheur Children's Hospital,
Memphis, Tennessee

TRE R. WELCH, PhD
Assistant Professor, Department of
Cardiovascular and Thoracic Surgery, The
University of Texas Southwestern Medical
Center, Dallas, Texas

JENNY E. ZABLAH, MD
Department of Pediatric Cardiology,
Children's Hospital of Colorado, University of
Colorado School of Medicine, Aurora,
Colorado

EVAN MICHAEL ZAHN, MD
Director, Guerin Family Congenital Heart
Program, Cedars-Sinai Medical Center, Los
Angeles, California

CONTENTS

Coarctation of the aorta is a common congenital heart defect and can present at any age. Infants may carry a fetal diagnosis, or are generally diagnosed after auscultation of a murmur, although rarely present in shock. Those that escape early childhood detection typically present in adolescence and adulthood, generally with upper-extremity hypertension. Percutaneous therapies have evolved to include balloon angioplasty and stent placement, and generally are the preferred first-line therapy for most adolescent/adult patients. Percutaneous interventions are now viable options in younger and smaller patients. The advent of bioresorbable stents may provide further expansion of treatment options to very small patients.

Patients with dysfunctional right ventricular outflow tracks comprise a large portion of patients with severe congenital heart disease. Transcatheter pulmonary valve replacement in patients with dysfunctional right ventricular outflow tracks is feasible, safe, and efficacious. This article reviews current transcatheter valve replacement technology for dysfunctional right ventricular outflow tract and pulmonary valvular disease and its applications to patients with congenital heart disease. Discussed are the approach and preprocedural planning, current options, and applications of transcatheter pulmonary valve therapy. Also considered are future directions in this field as the technologies begin to develop further.

Congenital heart defects that involve obstruction to the right ventricular outflow tract are common. Surgical repair involves early relief of right ventricular outflow tract obstruction, which typically results in pulmonary regurgitation and large irregularly shaped "native" right ventricular outflow tract. This type of anatomy represents the majority of patients who could potentially benefit from transcatheter pulmonary valve therapy. Currently approved balloon-expandable devices were not designed for this application and the unique anatomy of these patients presents tremendous challenges for designing a valve that is. This article explores those challenges and the newest self-expanding devices designed to treat this challenging population.

The quest for an ideal biodegradable stent for both adult coronary and pediatric congenital heart disease applications continues. Over the past few years, a lot of progress has been made toward development of a dedicated pediatric biodegradable stent that can be used for congenital heart disease applications. At present, there are no biodegradable stents available for use in congenital heart disease. In this article, the authors review the different biodegradable materials and their limitations and provide an overview of the current biodegradable stents being evaluated for congenital heart disease applications.

CONGENITAL HEART DISEASE INTERVENTION

RELATED SERIES

Cardiology Clinics
Cardiac Electrophysiology Clinics
Heart Failure Clinics

THE CLINICS ARE NOW AVAILABLE ONLINE!

Access your subscription at:
www.theclinics.com

PREFACE

Update in Congenital Interventions

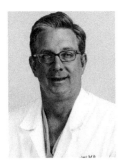

Daniel S. Levi, MD
Editor

The evolution in the world of interventional congenital heart disease has been driven by the availability of new and innovative devices over the past few decades. While originally, many of the devices and procedural techniques in congenital heart disease led to new procedures in structural heart disease, the constantly evolving world of structural heart disease is now contributing to advances in congenital heart disease. The massive investments in structural heart disease devices are trickling over to congenital interventions and allowing the smaller pediatric market access to devices like the Sapien valve designed originally for adults with calcific aortic stenosis.

Just 20 years ago, many doctors were skeptical that interventionalists would be able to regularly offer things like ventricular septal defect (VSD) closures and transcatheter pulmonary valve replacements. Currently, most atrial septal defects (ASDs), VSDs, coarctations, pulmonary artery stenoses, and even patent duct arteriosus (PDAs) in small babies are being treated in the cardiac catheterization lab rather than with surgery. Similarly, in many centers, nearly all pulmonary valve replacements are being treated without surgery.

The review articles in this issue cover basic interventions, more advanced interventions, and even devices that are still in preclinical development. This issue starts with articles on more basic and classic congenital interventions such as ASD closures, VSD closures, treatment of aortic coarctations, and pulmonary artery obstructions. The PDA article focuses on extension of PDA closure to small and even premature infants. The articles on transcatheter pulmonary valve replacements are separated into new uses of the classic balloon expandable valves and on the newer self-expanding valves. Both the article on bioresorbable stents and the article on self-expanding stents focus on many devices that remain in preclinical development.

We hope that this issue of *Interventional Cardiology Clinics* can provide a practical overview of the current state-of-the-art approach to common lesions found in both pediatric and adult congenital heart disease. We have asked many of the experts in congenital interventions to provide practical knowledge of basic interventions as well as reviews of devices that are certain to continue to revolutionize our field.

Daniel S. Levi, MD
UCLA Pediatrics
200 UCLA Medical Plaza, Suite 330
Los Angeles, CA 90095, USA

E-mail address:
dlevi@mednet.ucla.edu

Intervent Cardiol Clin 8 (2019) ix
https://doi.org/10.1016/j.iccl.2018.09.001
2211-7458/19/© 2018 Published by Elsevier Inc.

Ventricular Septal Defect Closure Devices, Techniques, and Outcomes

Brian H. Morray, MD

KEYWORDS

- Cardiac catheterization • Congenital heart disease • Pediatrics • Adult congenital heart disease
- Ventricular septal defect • Transcatheter VSD closure

KEY POINTS

- Early attempts at transcatheter ventricular septal defect (VSD) closure were successful but were associated with high complication rates in smaller patients, complete heart block, and residual shunts.
- The Amplatzer membranous VSD occluder experienced early success, but subsequent reports documented unacceptable rates of heart block and the device was not approved for use.
- The Amplatzer muscular VSD occluder was approved by the Food and Drug Administration in 2007 and is currently the only device approved for VSD closure in the United States.
- The development of additional devices and low-profile delivery systems has allowed for antegrade and retrograde closure of different VSD types with low complication rates and risk of heart block.

INTRODUCTION

Ventricular septal defects (VSDs) are a common form of congenital heart disease and can occur in isolation or in combination with other structural defects. They represent ~20% of all congenital heart lesions and are encountered in different positions within the ventricular septum. Large VSDs diagnosed prenatally or in infancy often result in signs of congestive heart failure and typically require surgical closure to ameliorate symptoms.

Smaller, more restrictive defects can remain relatively asymptomatic but can result in long-term sequelae such as pulmonary hypertension, left heart dilation, arrhythmia, aortic regurgitation, double chamber right ventricle, or endocarditis. Defects deemed hemodynamically significant (Qp:Qs >1.5:1) were traditionally closed by surgical means but presented an opportunity for transcatheter closure strategies.

The first published report of transcatheter VSD closure described 6 patients with a variety of VSD types who underwent closure with the Rashkind double umbrella device.[1] Following that initial description there were several reports documenting successful defect closure with a variety of devices including the Rashkind device, vascular coils, the buttoned device, and the Starflex device.[2–6] These early devices required large delivery sheaths and reported high rates of aortic and tricuspid valve damage and residual shunts.

More recently, transcatheter VSD closure using the family of vascular occlusion devices from Amplatzer (St. Jude Medical, St. Paul, MN, USA) has become increasingly common. Early reports using these devices documented a concerning incidence of complete heart block (CHB), particularly with membranous VSD closure. Recently, lower profile delivery systems

Disclosure Statement: No disclosures.

Division of Pediatric Cardiology, Seattle Children's Hospital, University of Washington School of Medicine, 4800 Sand Point Way Northeast, RC.2.820, Seattle, WA 98105, USA

E-mail address: brian.morray@seattlechildrens.org

https://doi.org/10.1016/j.iccl.2018.08.002
2211-7458/19/

and softer devices have improved success rates with lower rates of heart block and arrhythmia.

ANATOMY

VSDs are typically divided into 4 or 5 types with different nomenclature depending on the anatomic school of thought[7,8]:

- Atrioventricular canal type
- Muscular
- Membranous
- Conoventricular
- Conal septal or right ventricular outlet

Transcatheter closure of VSDs is typically reserved for membranous or muscular defects although there are reports of successful transcatheter closure of conal septal defects. Atrioventricular canal type defects are typically seen with common AV canal defects or inlet VSDs. Conoventricular VSDs typically occur in combination with hypoplasia or malalignment of the conal septum as seen in tetralogy of Fallot (anterior malalignment) or interrupted aortic arch (posterior malalignment).

INDICATIONS AND CONTRAINDICATIONS

Large VSDs diagnosed prenatally or early in infancy either alone or in combination with other congenital heart defects often result in pulmonary overcirculation and symptoms of congestive heart failure with early failure to thrive. These defects are typically closed surgically. Transcatheter VSD closure is typically performed outside of the neonatal period when there is evidence of a hemodynamically significant shunt. Indications for transcatheter VSD closure include the following:

- Cardiomegaly or left heart dilation by echocardiogram
- Qp:Qs greater than 1.5
- Failure to thrive
- Worsening New York Heart Association class symptoms
- Recurrent respiratory infections
- History of infective endocarditis

Acute onset left to right shunting as occurs in the setting of septal rupture following myocardial infarction can result in severe pulmonary overcirculation with pulmonary edema and cardiogenic shock with end-organ dysfunction.

With the earlier generations of devices the delivery systems were large and small patient size was often considered a contraindication. With the development of low-profile delivery systems, small devices, and hybrid approaches to vascular access such as the perventricular approach, smaller patients are able to undergo transcatheter device closure. Typical contraindications for device closure include the following:

- Irreversible pulmonary vascular disease (>7 U/m^2)
- Contraindication to antiplatelet therapy
- Active infection or sepsis
- Anatomic concerns
  - Inadequate rim (<2 mm) below the aortic valve in a membranous VSD
  - Supracristal defects
  - Aortic valve cusp prolapse
  - Malalignment VSDs (associated with tetralogy of Fallot or other conotruncal defects)

PROCEDURE

The procedural steps for device closure have been well documented. The approach to closure is dictated by patient and defect size, defect location, and history of vascular occlusions. In the early studies of transcatheter VSD closure, an antegrade approach was typically used, which involved the creation of an arteriovenous wire loop and delivery of the device from a venous approach. With the development of low-profile delivery systems a retrograde approach from the femoral artery is increasingly used and obviates the need for a wire loop (Fig. 1). In smaller patients or those with VSDs that are difficult to access, a perventricular approach through a full or limited sternotomy can be effective (Fig. 2).

An initial hemodynamic assessment should be performed to document the size of the shunt and evaluate for the presence of pulmonary hypertension. Any evidence of elevated pulmonary vascular resistance (PVR) should prompt vasodilator studies to determine if the elevated PVR is reversible. If the patient is an appropriate hemodynamic candidate for device closure, careful angiographic and echocardiographic assessment of the defect is important. A left ventricular (LV) angiogram in a long axial oblique projection (LAO 60°, CRA 30°) will profile the size and number of any defects, the relationship of a membranous defect to the aortic valve, and the presence of any aneurysmal or obstructive tissue on the right ventricular (RV) side (Fig. 3). Adjunctive echocardiographic imaging is also important for assessment before, during, and after device placement. Transesophageal echocardiography (TEE) is the most common mode of imaging

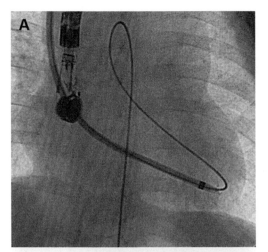

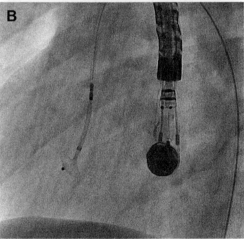

Fig. 1. (A) An arteriovenous wire loop is established from the femoral artery retrograde into the left ventricle and across the ventricular septal defect into the right ventricle and up to the right internal jugular vein (RIJV). The sheath is advanced antegrade from RIJV across the defect to deliver the device. (B) A retrograde approach directly from the femoral artery, across the aortic valve and directly across the VSD into the right ventricle.

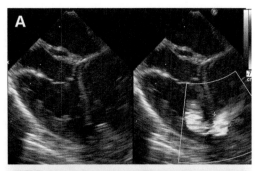

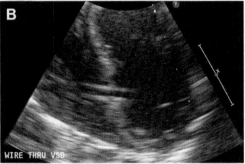

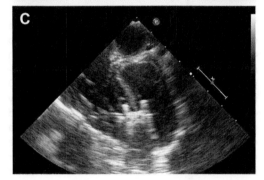

Fig. 2. Perventricular closure of a large apical muscular VSD in a 4-month-old boy (A). Intraoperative TEE imaging demonstrates the defect and guides the passage of the wire and sheath from the RV free wall through the defect and into the LV (B). An Amplatzer muscular VSD occluder is deployed through the sheath and position is confirmed with TEE before release (C). LV, left ventricle; RV, right ventricular; TEE, transesophageal echocardiogram. (Courtesy of Abbott, Inc, St Paul, MN.)

used in device closures although the use of intracardiac echocardiography has been described.

Antegrade Approach

An antegrade approach is the more commonly described technique and typically requires the creation of an arteriovenous wire loop to advance the delivery system. This technique can be used to close membranous, muscular, and postsurgical residual defects and postinfarction VSDs. The VSD is crossed from the LV side using a right coronary diagnostic catheter or guide and a floppy tipped guidewire. The wire is exchanged for a 0.035″ exchange length guidewire, which is then snared in the pulmonary artery or superior vena cava and externalized through the femoral venous sheath, creating an arteriovenous wire loop. The delivery sheath is advanced over the wire from the vein (femoral, internal jugular, or hepatic), across the defect and into the ascending aorta. The device is often partially advanced beyond the tip of the delivery sheath in the ascending aorta in order to avoid damage to the aortic valve as the sheath is withdrawn into the LV. The device can then be deployed and released under echocardiographic guidance.

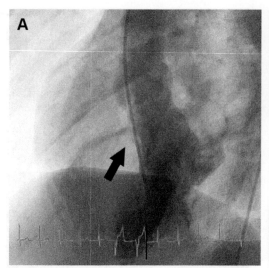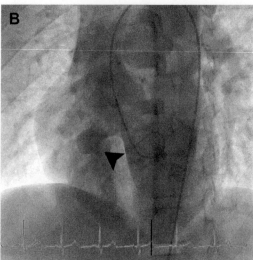

Fig. 3. (A) LV angiogram in a long axial oblique projection demonstrates a membranous VSD (*arrow*) without restrictive tissue on the RV side. (B) In a similar projection, LV angiography demonstrates a prominent aneurysm or "wind-sock" of tissue (*arrowhead*), partially obstructing the defect on the RV side.

Retrograde Approach

The retrograde approach involves closure of the defect from the arterial side without the need to create an arteriovenous loop.[9,10] This approach is increasingly used in the current era of lower-profile delivery catheters and devices. The VSD is crossed from the LV side using a right coronary diagnostic catheter or guide and a floppy tipped guidewire. The catheter can be exchanged for a delivery sheath or the coronary guide can be used to deploy the device. The delivery catheter is advanced into the RV and the device is partially deployed on the RV side before complete deployment across the defect. The proposed advantages of the retrograde approach are shorter procedural times and decreased risk of conduction disturbances or heart block. This approach generally does decrease procedural times but there are insufficient data and no comparative trials documenting differences in heart block risk between the antegrade and retrograde techniques.

Hybrid Approach

Muscular VSDs in small children can be difficult to close surgically due to poor direct visualization of the defects.[11] This can result in significant residual defects. Percutaneous closure of these types of defects can also be limited due to hemodynamic instability related to large sheath manipulation in a small patient. Direct perventricular puncture of the RV free wall can greatly improve the access to the defect and allow for placement of large devices. This approach was

first described in 1998 and more recently in a multicenter study of 47 patients.[12,13] Through a full or limited sternotomy a purse string suture is placed and the RV free wall is punctured. Using TEE or epicardial echo guidance a wire can be advanced directly across the defect into the LV and an appropriately sized sheath advanced over the wire. With the sheath in the LV, an appropriately sized device can be deployed under echocardiographic guidance. Following deployment the sheath is removed and the purse string suture tied down to manage bleeding.

DEVICES AND OUTCOMES

A variety of different devices have been used in the past for transcatheter VSD closure, including the Rashkind double umbrella device, vascular coils, the buttoned device, and the Starflex device. These devices were used in an off-label fashion to close a variety of different VSD types.

Amplatzer Membranous Ventricular Septal Defect Occluder

In the early 2000s the Amplatzer membranous and muscular VSD occluders became available (Fig. 4). The US phase 1 trial of the membranous device published in 2003 documented successful closure rates of 91% with complete defect closure in 96% of patients at 6-month follow-up and only 1 case of CHB.[14] These results were mirrored by other small studies that demonstrated high procedural success rates and

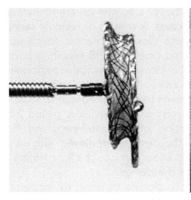
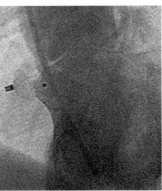
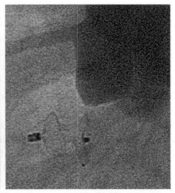

Fig. 4. The asymmetric shape of the Amplatzer membranous VSD occluder, designed to sit across the defect without distorting the aortic valve. LV and aortic root angiograms demonstrate complete closure of the defect without impinging on the aortic valve. A radiopaque marker on the LV disk helped to confirm appropriate device position. (*Courtesy of* Abbott, Inc, St Paul, MN; and *Adapted from* Bass JL, Kalra GS, Arora R, et al. Initial human experience with the Amplatzer perimembranous ventricular septal occluder device. Catheter Cardiovasc Interv 2003;58(2):238–45; with permission.)

closure rates greater than 95% with rare cases of CHB.[15,16] Following these initial reports, additional studies began to demonstrate higher rates of CHB, ranging from 2% to 22%.[17–20] Cases of CHB requiring pacemaker implantation were reported months after device placement and often without any preceding changes in symptoms or electrocardiogram (ECG). Risk factors for the development of CHB were difficult to elucidate, although in a study that described a higher rate of CHB, the patients were significantly smaller compared with prior studies.[20] Given the concerns over conduction disturbances, particularly remote from the time of placement, the Amplatzer membranous VSD occluder was not approved for use and is no longer clinically available. The Amplatzer membranous VSD occluder II was designed to prevent conduction abnormalities by reducing radial force and increasing

device stability. A small study of 19 patients described successful closure of the defect in 95% of cases with no increase in aortic or tricuspid valve regurgitation and no instances of CHB requiring pacemaker at 1-year follow-up.[21]

Amplatzer Muscular Ventricular Septal Defect Occluder

Use of the Amplatzer muscular VSD occluder was first reported in an animal model in 1999 (**Fig. 5**).[22] This was followed by a series of small clinical reports documenting high rates of successful closure.[23,24] The results of attempted closure in 75 patients enrolled as part of a multicenter registry were published in 2004.[25] The procedure was successful in 85% of patients. Most of the devices were deployed using an antegrade approach from the RV. Major adverse

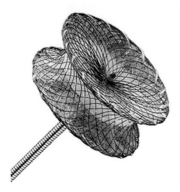
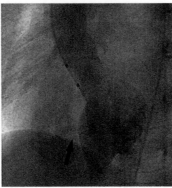
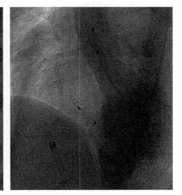

Fig. 5. The Amplatzer muscular VSD occluder has 2 symmetric disks with a central waist. LV angiogram in a long axial oblique projection demonstrates a midmuscular VSD (*arrow*). After establishing an arteriovenous wire loop the device is deployed across the defect. LV angiography confirms complete closure of the defect. (*Courtesy of* Abbott, Inc, St Paul, MN.)

events were documented in 10% of cases with 2 procedure-related deaths. Conduction abnormalities or arrhythmia were described in 20% of cases but there were no cases of CHB requiring pacemaker placement. Immediately following the procedure, there was complete defect closure in 47% of cases, which increased to 92% at the 12-month follow-up. Lower patient weight at the time of procedure (<5 kg) was significantly correlated with procedural complications and the presence of a post procedure residual shunt. The muscular VSD occluder was approved for use by the Food and Drug Administration in 2007. The muscular VSD occluder has also been used to close membranous and post-myocardial infarction VSDs.[10,26,27]

Amplatzer Duct Occluder I and II

Both the Amplatzer duct occluder (ADO) I and II devices have been used in an off-label fashion to close membranous, muscular, and residual post-surgical VSDs (Fig. 6). The ADO I has been used to close membranous VSDs with redundant tricuspid valve tissue or a "wind-sock" aneurysm

formation on the RV side with greater than 90% procedural success, low rates of residual shunts (>95% complete closure at recent follow-up), and no reported cases of CHB requiring pacemaker.[28,29] The closure is typically performed by creating an arteriovenous loop and advancing the delivery sheath from an antegrade approach. The retention disc of the device is pulled into the wide portion of the aneurysm, and the remainder of the device is deployed within the opening of the aneurysm into the RV creating a slight waist on the device.

Transcatheter closure of small to moderate membranous and muscular VSDs with the ADO II has more recently been described. The device uses a low-profile delivery sheath that allows for retrograde arterial deployment. Recent published series have described procedural success rates greater than 90% with complete closure rates approaching 95% at recent follow-up and only rare cases of permanent conduction abnormalities.[9,30–32] The device is typically sized 1 to 2 mm greater than the diameter of the defect. The largest ADO II has a waist diameter of

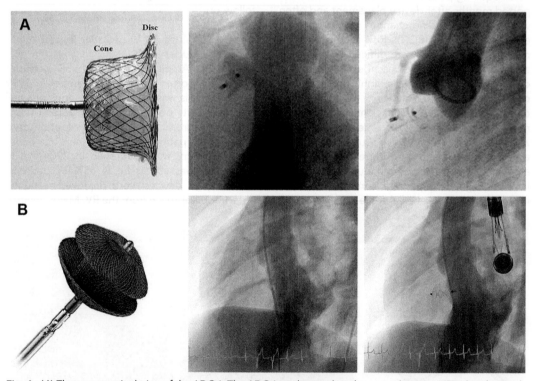

Fig. 6. (A) The asymmetric design of the ADO I. The ADO I can be used to close membranous VSDs by placing the device completely within the aneurysm on the RV side without impinging on the rims of the defect or the aortic valve as demonstrated in these LV and aortic root angiograms. (B) The symmetric ADO II has been used to close membranous and muscular VSDs from both a retrograde and an antegrade approach. ([A, B] Courtesy of Abbott, Inc, St Paul, MN; and [A] Adapted from El Said HG, Bratincsak A, Gordon BM, et al. Closure of perimembranous ventricular septal defects with aneurysmal tissue using the Amplazter Duct Occluder I: lessons learned and medium term follow up. Catheter Cardiovasc Interv 2012;80(6):900; with permission.)

6 mm, which limits the size of the defect that can be closed to typically less than 6 mm. In addition, the diameters of the retention discs are 6 mm larger than the waist, so there has to be adequate distance from the superior edge of the defect to the aortic valve (typically >2–3 mm).

Nit-Occlud Coil

The PFM Nit-Occlud VSD coil is designed for membranous and muscular VSD closure and received a CE mark in 2010 for dedicated VSD closure (**Fig. 7**). The device is a nitinol coil with attached polyester fibers and has an asymmetric design with a larger left-sided cone and a smaller right-sided cone. It comes in multiple sizes and can be implanted in VSDs with and without restrictive aneurysmal tissue. In a multicenter European registry, the device was successfully implanted in 92% of cases.[33] Procedural failure occurred in 8% of cases related to device to defect mismatch, transient heart block, aortic valve impingement, large residual shunt, and improper device positioning. Hemolysis occurred in almost 4% of cases (4 patients) with spontaneous resolution in 2 patients, placement of a second device in 1 patient, and surgical removal and VSD closure in 1 patient. Device embolization occurred in 1 case and required surgical removal of the device. There was 1 case of CHB following device placement that resolved with a course of steroids. There were no instances of conduction abnormalities requiring surgical removal of the device or pacemaker implantation. Complete closure was achieved in 99% of cases at most recent follow-up.

Additional Devices

The Cera family of VSD occluders (Lifetech, Shenzhen, China) are available outside of the United States for closure of membranous, muscular, and postinfarction VSDs. The Cera devices have a self-expanding nitinol frame and are available in 3 different designs (2 symmetric and 1 asymmetric). In a multicenter study of 55 patients, the procedural success rate was 91%. There was 1 case of device embolization that was retrieved percutaneously. CHB developed in 1 patient requiring a pacemaker, and 1 patient developed aortic regurgitation requiring surgical device removal.[34] Complete closure of the defect was documented in 91% of patients at recent follow-up.

The Occlutech membranous and muscular VSD occluders (Helsingborg, Sweden) are self-expanding nitinol-based devices and are available for use outside of the United States. There are limited reports of these products in the medical literature.

ADVERSE EVENTS

Conduction Abnormalities

Conduction disturbances remain an area of concern, particularly following membranous VSD closure given the proximity of the conduction system to the defect. The proposed mechanism is the exertion of radial force from the device, resulting in injury to the surrounding tissue including the conduction system. Early studies of the Amplatzer membranous VSD occluder documented CHB rates of 2% to 22% and ultimately that device was not approved for clinical use.[17–20] Of particular concern was the development of CHB months to years

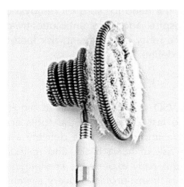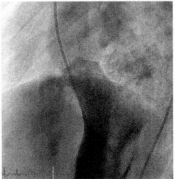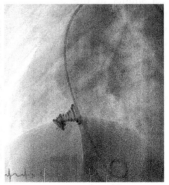

Fig. 7. The Nit-Occlud VSD coil has an asymmetric design with a larger coil segment on the LV side. The device sits across the membranous defect anchored in place by the larger coil on the LV side. (*Courtesy of* PFM Medical, Inc., Carlsbad, CA; and *Adapted from* Haas NA, Kock L, Bertram H, et al. Interventional VSD-closure with the Nit-Occlud((R)) Le VSD-coil in 110 patients: early and midterm results of the EUREVECO-registry. Pediatr Cardiol 2017;38(2):220; with permission.)

following implant, which was described in several studies.[17,35] Risk factors for CHB and pacemaker implantation have been difficult to define. In a multicenter European registry of transcatheter VSD closure, univariate analysis identified the use of the Amplatzer membranous VSD occluder and VSD location as risk factors for CHB although these were not significant in the multivariate analysis.[18] Smaller patient size and device oversizing have been proposed as additional risk factors.[17] A study of 228 subjects implanted with either the Amplatzer membranous VSD occluder or the Lifetech symmetric VSD occluder demonstrated that defects farther from the aortic valve and closer to the tricuspid valve were at greater risk of developing CHB, suggesting that defect position and its relationship to the conduction system play a role in the development of CHB.[35]

More recent studies of the ADO I and II and the Nit-Occlud coil have demonstrated lower rates of CHB, typically less than 2% of cases.[9,28–33] Although conduction abnormalities have been described in the closure of muscular VSDs, this complication is less common. The successful use of steroids has been reported in various case series as a treatment for device-related CHB although no larger studies have been performed.[35,36] The prophylactic use of steroids in these patients has been studied but not in a placebo-controlled fashion, and this practice has not been widely adopted by most centers.[37]

Residual Shunt

Based on the width of the color doppler jet around the device, residual shunts are typically defined as trivial (<1 mm), small (1–2 mm), moderate (2–4 mm), and large (>4 mm). Large residual shunts at the time of implant have been reported and typically result in immediate device removal and subsequent placement of a larger device or surgical referral. For most contemporary devices and techniques, complete closure rates are greater than 90% at recent follow-up.[9,17,28] Surgical removal of a device for severe residual shunt has been rarely reported.[18,29]

Aortic Valve Distortion

Distortion of the aortic valve related to the device closure of membranous VSDs was described in up to 9% of patients early in the experience with the Amplatzer membranous VSD occluder and has been described with other devices.[19] This is often recognized during the procedure with careful echocardiographic imaging and

the device is removed before release. Aortic regurgitation following device implant is typically mild and rarely results in the need for device removal. Care should be taken to evaluate the distance between the defect and the aortic valve. In most studies a distance greater than 2 mm is considered acceptable although this distance may need to be greater with symmetric devices such as the ADO II or Amplatzer muscular VSD occluder. Device placement within aneurysmal tissue on the RV side can potentially reduce the risk to the aortic valve by increasing the distance from the device to the valve.[28,29]

Hemolysis

Hemolysis has been reported in 1% to 2% of cases in most large studies and across different device types. Cases are typically mild and resolve spontaneously within 2 to 3 days of implant. The need for blood transfusion or surgical removal of the device is rare.[18,28] Risk factors for hemolysis following device closure have been difficult to define.

Device Embolization

Device embolization has also been reported in 1% to 2% of cases and across different device types. Embolization typically occurs shortly after device deployment or within 24 hours of the case, and the device can be retrieved in the catheterization laboratory. The need for surgical removal of an embolized device is rare.

Endocarditis

Endocarditis following transcatheter VSD closure is rare. There are only a few case reports documenting infection specifically related to the device. Cases have been described with multiple device types and with and without any residual VSD.[38–40] This is a serious complication because it can result in the need for surgical removal of the device despite adequate antibiotic treatment. Given the rarity of this event, risk factors are difficult to define.

SUMMARY

Transcatheter VSD closure has evolved significantly over the last 20 years as the tools and techniques have improved. Large delivery systems and the risk of heart block and residual shunts made the early experience challenging. The evolution of lower-profile delivery systems and the off-label use of additional devices have made the procedure safer and more effective. Still, there is only 1 device approved in the United States for transcatheter VSD closure. In the current era, adverse event rates are low.

Despite these improvements, the risk of adverse events, particularly serious conduction abnormalities, remain and the need for careful technique and patient selection is important. The development of novel devices designed for transcatheter VSD closure will continue to advance the success of this procedure going forward.

REFERENCES

1. Lock JE, Block PC, McKay RG, et al. Transcatheter closure of ventricular septal defects. Circulation 1988;78(2):361–8.
2. Rigby ML, Redington AN. Primary transcatheter umbrella closure of perimembranous ventricular septal defect. Br Heart J 1994;72(4):368–71.
3. Kalra GS, Verma PK, Dhall A, et al. Transcatheter device closure of ventricular septal defects: immediate results and intermediate-term follow-up. Am Heart J 1999;138(2 Pt 1):339–44.
4. Kalra GS, Verma PK, Singh S, et al. Transcatheter closure of ventricular septal defect using detachable steel coil. Heart 1999;82(3):395–6.
5. Sideris EB, Walsh KP, Haddad JL, et al. Occlusion of congenital ventricular septal defects by the buttoned device. "Buttoned device" Clinical Trials International Register. Heart 1997;77(3):276–9.
6. Knauth AL, Lock JE, Perry SB, et al. Transcatheter device closure of congenital and postoperative residual ventricular septal defects. Circulation 2004;110(5):501–7.
7. Van Praagh R, Geva T, Kreutzer J. Ventricular septal defects: how shall we describe, name and classify them? J Am Coll Cardiol 1989;14(5):1298–9.
8. Soto B, Ceballos R, Kirklin JW. Ventricular septal defects: a surgical viewpoint. J Am Coll Cardiol 1989;14(5):1291–7.
9. Koneti NR, Sreeram N, Penumatsa RR, et al. Transcatheter retrograde closure of perimembranous ventricular septal defects in children with the Amplatzer duct occluder II device. J Am Coll Cardiol 2012;60(23):2421–2.
10. Muthusamy K. Retrograde closure of perimembranous ventricular septal defect using muscular ventricular septal occluder: a single-center experience of a novel technique. Pediatr Cardiol 2015;36(1):106–10.
11. Michel-Behnke I, Ewert P, Koch A, et al. Device closure of ventricular septal defects by hybrid procedures: a multicenter retrospective study. Catheter Cardiovasc Interv 2011;77(2):242–51.
12. Amin Z, Berry JM, Foker JE, et al. Intraoperative closure of muscular ventricular septal defect in a canine model and application of the technique in a baby. J Thorac Cardiovasc Surg 1998;115(6):1374–6.
13. Gray RG, Menon SC, Johnson JT, et al. Acute and midterm results following perventricular device closure of muscular ventricular septal defects: a multicenter PICES investigation. Catheter Cardiovasc Interv 2017;90(2):281–9.
14. Fu YC, Bass J, Amin Z, et al. Transcatheter closure of perimembranous ventricular septal defects using the new Amplatzer membranous VSD occluder: results of the U.S. phase I trial. J Am Coll Cardiol 2006;47(2):319–25.
15. Hijazi ZM, Hakim F, Haweleh AA, et al. Catheter closure of perimembranous ventricular septal defects using the new Amplatzer membranous VSD occluder: initial clinical experience. Catheter Cardiovasc Interv 2002;56(4):508–15.
16. Bass JL, Kalra GS, Arora R, et al. Initial human experience with the Amplatzer perimembranous ventricular septal occluder device. Catheter Cardiovasc Interv 2003;58(2):238–45.
17. Butera G, Carminati M, Chessa M, et al. Transcatheter closure of perimembranous ventricular septal defects: early and long-term results. J Am Coll Cardiol 2007;50(12):1189–95.
18. Carminati M, Butera G, Chessa M, et al. Transcatheter closure of congenital ventricular septal defects: results of the European Registry. Eur Heart J 2007;28(19):2361–8.
19. Holzer R, de Giovanni J, Walsh KP, et al. Transcatheter closure of perimembranous ventricular septal defects using the amplatzer membranous VSD occluder: immediate and midterm results of an international registry. Catheter Cardiovasc Interv 2006;68(4):620–8.
20. Predescu D, Chaturvedi RR, Friedberg MK, et al. Complete heart block associated with device closure of perimembranous ventricular septal defects. J Thorac Cardiovasc Surg 2008;136(5):1223–8.
21. Tzikas A, Ibrahim R, Velasco-Sanchez D, et al. Transcatheter closure of perimembranous ventricular septal defect with the Amplatzer((R)) membranous VSD occluder 2: initial world experience and one-year follow-up. Catheter Cardiovasc Interv 2014;83(4):571–80.
22. Amin Z, Gu X, Berry JM, et al. New device for closure of muscular ventricular septal defects in a canine model. Circulation 1999;100(3):320–8.
23. Thanopoulos BD, Tsaousis GS, Konstadopoulou GN, et al. Transcatheter closure of muscular ventricular septal defects with the amplatzer ventricular septal defect occluder: initial clinical applications in children. J Am Coll Cardiol 1999;33(5):1395–9.
24. Hijazi ZM, Hakim F, Al-Fadley F, et al. Transcatheter closure of single muscular ventricular septal defects using the amplatzer muscular VSD occluder: initial results and technical considerations. Catheter Cardiovasc Interv 2000;49(2):167–72.

25. Holzer R, Balzer D, Cao QL, et al. Device closure of muscular ventricular septal defects using the Amplatzer muscular ventricular septal defect occluder: immediate and mid-term results of a U.S. registry. J Am Coll Cardiol 2004;43(7):1257–63.
26. Holzer R, Balzer D, Amin Z, et al. Transcatheter closure of postinfarction ventricular septal defects using the new Amplatzer muscular VSD occluder: results of a U.S. Registry. Catheter Cardiovasc Interv 2004;61(2):196–201.
27. Egbe AC, Poterucha JT, Rihal CS, et al. Transcatheter closure of postmyocardial infarction, iatrogenic, and postoperative ventricular septal defects: the Mayo Clinic experience. Catheter Cardiovasc Interv 2015;86(7):1264–70.
28. El Said HG, Bratincsak A, Gordon BM, et al. Closure of perimembranous ventricular septal defects with aneurysmal tissue using the Amplazter Duct Occluder I: lessons learned and medium term follow up. Catheter Cardiovasc Interv 2012;80(6):895–903.
29. Landman G, Kipps A, Moore P, et al. Outcomes of a modified approach to transcatheter closure of perimembranous ventricular septal defects. Catheter Cardiovasc Interv 2013;82(1):143–9.
30. El-Sisi A, Sobhy R, Jaccoub V, et al. Perimembranous ventricular septal defect device closure: choosing between amplatzer duct occluder I and II. Pediatr Cardiol 2017;38(3):596–602.
31. Ghosh S, Sridhar A, Sivaprakasam M. Complete heart block following transcatheter closure of perimembranous VSD using amplatzer duct occluder II. Catheter Cardiovasc Interv 2017. [Epub ahead of print].
32. Narin N, Pamukcu O, Tuncay A, et al. Percutaneous ventricular septal defect closure in patients under 1 year of age. Pediatr Cardiol 2018;39(5):1009–15.
33. Haas NA, Kock L, Bertram H, et al. Interventional VSD-closure with the Nit-Occlud((R)) Le VSD-coil in 110 patients: early and midterm results of the EUREVECO-registry. Pediatr Cardiol 2017;38(2):215–27.
34. Esteves CA, Solarewicz LA, Cassar R, et al. Occlusion of the perimembranous ventricular septal defect using CERA(R) devices. Catheter Cardiovasc Interv 2012;80(2):182–7.
35. Yang R, Kong XQ, Sheng YH, et al. Risk factors and outcomes of post-procedure heart blocks after transcatheter device closure of perimembranous ventricular septal defect. JACC Cardiovasc Interv 2012;5(4):422–7.
36. Yip WC, Zimmerman F, Hijazi ZM. Heart block and empirical therapy after transcatheter closure of perimembranous ventricular septal defect. Catheter Cardiovasc Interv 2005;66(3):436–41.
37. Thakkar B, Patel N, Bohora S, et al. Transcatheter device closure of perimembranous ventricular septal defect in children treated with prophylactic oral steroids: acute and mid-term results of a single-centre, prospective, observational study. Cardiol Young 2016;26(4):669–76.
38. El-Sisi AM, Menaissy YM, Bekheet SA. Infective endocarditis following coil occlusion of perimembranous ventricular septal defect with the Nit-Occlud(((R))) Le device. Ann Pediatr Cardiol 2016;9(1):59–61.
39. Kassis I, Shachor-Meyouhas Y, Khatib I, et al. Kingella endocarditis after closure of ventricular septal defect with a transcatheter device. Pediatr Infect Dis J 2012;31(1):105–6.
40. Scheuerman O, Bruckheimer E, Marcus N, et al. Endocarditis after closure of ventricular septal defect by transcatheter device. Pediatrics 2006;117(6):e1256–8.

State-of-the-Art Atrial Septal Defect Closure Devices for Congenital Heart

Michael L. O'Byrne, MD, MSCE[a],*, Daniel S. Levi, MD[b]

KEYWORDS

• Erosion • Pediatric cardiology • Transcatheter intervention • Outcomes

KEY POINTS

- Transcatheter device closure of ostium secundum atrial defects (ASD) has a lower risk of mortality and morbidity, shorter length of stay, and lower cost than operative closure of the same defect.
- Erosion of devices after transcatheter closure of ASD remains an important consideration in transcatheter closure of ASD. The best data to date indicate that patients with erosion were more likely than control subjects to have smaller superior rims, larger defects relative to the septum and patient size, and were more likely to have an oversized device. Although these findings suggest steps that might improve outcomes, further research is necessary to determine whether a specific subset of patients can be identified whose risk of device erosion exceeds the risks of open heart surgery.
- Transcatheter ASD closure remains the predominant method of ASD closure in children and young adults, but in recent years (coincident with concern for device erosion) there is a significant trend toward increasing referral for operative ASD closure. Simultaneously, the patient population referred for ASD closure is progressively younger with time. The effect of these trends on outcomes is not clear at this time, but deserves attention.
- Recent data have demonstrated the benefit of device closure of PFO as secondary prophylaxis for strokes in older adults. There is a dearth of data regarding the relative risks and benefits of this practice in younger patients with cryptogenic stroke and PFO. Given the high prevalence of PFO and increasing incidence of stroke in medically complicated pediatric patients, closure of PFO for this indication is likely to be an increasingly important issue for pediatric/congenital cardiologists.
- A potential innovation in closure of ASD and PFO are approaches that avoid implantation of a permanent device. An example is catheter-delivered sutures to close atrial defects, such as the NobleStitch device.

Conflicts of Interest: Dr M.L. O'Byrne has no significant conflicts to disclose. Dr D.S. Levi has no conflicts to disclose.
Funding Sources: Dr M.L. O'Byrne receives research support from the National Institute of Health/National Heart, Lung, and Blood Institute (K23 HL130420-01). The funding agencies had no role in the drafting of the manuscript or influencing its content. This article represents the opinion of the authors alone. There are no other relevant financial disclosures.
[a] Division of Cardiology, Department of Pediatrics, The Children's Hospital of Philadelphia, Perelman School of Medicine at the University of Pennsylvania, Center for Pediatric Clinical Effectiveness, Leonard Davis Institute, University of Pennsylvania, 34th Street and Civic Center Boulevard, Philadelphia, PA 19104, USA; [b] Division of Cardiology, UCLA Mattel Children's Hospital, University of California Los Angeles Medical School, 200 UCLA Medical Plaza #330, Los Angeles, CA 90095, USA
* Corresponding author.
E-mail address: obyrnem@email.chop.edu

Intervent Cardiol Clin 8 (2019) 11–21
https://doi.org/10.1016/j.iccl.2018.08.008
2211-7458/19/© 2018 Elsevier Inc. All rights reserved.

CURRENT DEVICES FOR TRANSCATHETER CLOSURE OF ATRIAL SEPTAL DEFECTS

With an incidence of 6 to 10 per 10,000 live births,[1] ostium secundum atrial septal defects (ASD) are one of the most common forms of congenital heart disease. King and Mills developed the first device for transcatheter closure of ASD (TC-ASD) in 1976.[2] The history of device development for TC-ASD is a testament to innovation in congenital/structural cardiology.[3] Over time, TC-ASD has become the predominant technique for closing most ASD; greater than 80% of isolated ASD treated at primary pediatric hospitals in the United States are closed in the catheterization laboratory.[4]

Two devices for TC-ASD are widely available in the United States (Fig. 1): the Amplatzer septal occluder (ASO) (St. Jude Medical, St. Paul, MN) (see Fig. 1A; Fig. 2) and the Gore Cardioform device (W.L. Gore and Associates, Flagstaff, AZ) (see Fig. 1B). The ASO was the first device approved by the Food and Drug Administration for TC-ASD demonstrating safety and efficacy in a nonrandomized IDE (Investigational Drug Exemption) trial,[5] which was reinforced in a subsequent multicenter registry study.[6] It has been in use long enough for several large single-center case series to report excellent medium- and long-term outcomes.[7–9] In contemporary case series of US centers, the ASO is used in between 70% and 86% of cases.[4,10]

The Gore Helex septal occluder (W.L. Gore and Associates) has also demonstrated excellent safety and efficacy in short-[11–13] and middle-term outcomes.[14] The Helex septal occluder has been replaced by the Gore Cardioform device and is no longer sold in the United States. The Cardioform device has a Nitinol wire frame covered with an expanded tetrafluoroethylene membrane. Like the Helex before it, this device was not self-centering and limited to small defects. The initial device trial and continuing access series are complete with manuscripts pending at this time. Gore has produced a second Cardioform device, the Cardioform atrial septal defect occluder, with a larger diameter central waist and an expanded range of diameters, both designed to facilitate closure of larger diameter ASDs (see Fig. 1C; Fig. 3). The newer Cardioform atrial septal defect occluder device is currently undergoing a Food and Drug Administration Pivotal trial (Gore ASSURED Trial; Clinical Trials.gov Identifier NCT02985684) in the United States. In a multicenter series from Canada, both Gore devices have demonstrated similar safety and efficacy to previous devices.[15] The Amplatzer multifenestrated septal occluder (Cribriform device; St. Jude Medical) resembles the ASO device but has symmetric discs and a narrow waist, designed to allow it to cover the septum of patients with multiple defects.

DEVICE EROSION OF THE AMPLATZER SEPTAL OCCLUDER DEVICE

Erosions of the device following TC-ASD with the Amplatzer device were first reported in a series of case reports in 2003 and 2004.[16–18] Alarm about erosions was particularly acute because of the perception that TC-ASD was technically straightforward and demonstrably safer than operative open heart surgical ASD (O-ASD), the catastrophic potential of erosions, and erosions seemed to occur unpredictably and years after device implantation. Rapidly, a board of physicians was convened to review known cases of device erosion, identifying deficient anterior-superior or retroaortic rim (along with device oversizing) as a risk factor present in all of their cases.[19] In 2012, a US Food and Drug Administration Panel Review convened and was followed by revision of the manufacturer's Indication for Use, labeling a retroaortic rim less than 5 mm in diameter as a relative contraindication to TC-ASD with an ASO device.[20–22] Concern for device erosion has persisted,[23–27] but limitations in longitudinal follow-up of implanted devices has made it impossible to accurately measure the number of devices implanted, the total number of erosions, and the risk of erosion. Best estimates of risk are between 0.04% and 0.3% of device implants.[19,21,23,24,28] Most cases of erosion occur shortly after device implantation, but erosions have been reported as late as 8 years after initial placement.[29,30]

The low overall rates of erosion and limited experience at individual centers has complicated identification of patient- and procedure-level risk factors for device erosion. Neither the first version of the IMPACT[4] nor C3PO[10] contained data about postdischarge adverse events. Since that time, a prospective postmarket surveillance study of the ASO was initiated. However, enrollment was stopped in December of 2016, and the results have yet to be published. In the first revision of the IMPACT registry the capacity to include follow-up data for prespecified interventions including TC-ASD was added. It remains to be seen whether centers are accurately reporting their longitudinal data in this voluntary database. Without manufacturer or registry follow-up, use of other large (nonclinical) observational

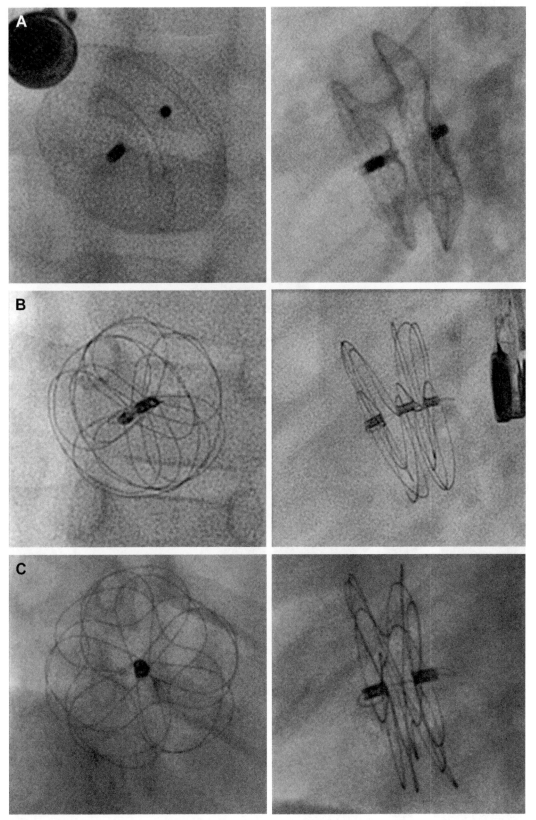

Fig. 1. Radiographic appearance of devices for transcatheter closure of ASD. Digital acquisition images of (A) Amplatzer septal occluder (anterior posterior and lateral projections), (B) Gore Cardioform device (en face and orthogonal views), and (C) Cardioform atrial septal defect occluder (en face and orthogonal views). (*Courtesy of* [A] Abbott, Inc, Abbott Park, IL, with permission; [B] GORE® CARDIOFORM Septal Occluder; and [C] GORE® CARDIOFORM Septal Occluder.)

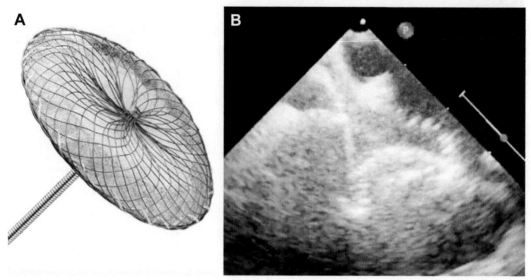

Fig. 2. (*A*) Amplatzer septal occluder (artist rendition). (*B*) Echocardiographic appearance of the Amplatzer ASD device splayed around the aorta. (*Courtesy of* [A] Abbott Laboratories, IL; and [B] Abbott, Inc, Abbott Park, IL; with permission.)

data-sets (eg, insurance claims data) may be necessary to obtain better estimates of erosion risk in the current era.

At present, it remains up to individual cardiologists to determine whether TC-ASD is the best option for ASD closure. There are not, as of yet, data to determine whether anatomic variations (bare vs small retroaortic rim or concomitant deficient superior tissue rim) or a combination of anatomy and choice of device (a patient with deficient retroaortic or superior rim and a large or oversized device) can provide superior risk stratification.[19,28,31] Although deficient retroaortic rim has consistently been found in erosion cases, it is not sufficient to identify which patients are at risk for erosion. Subsequent

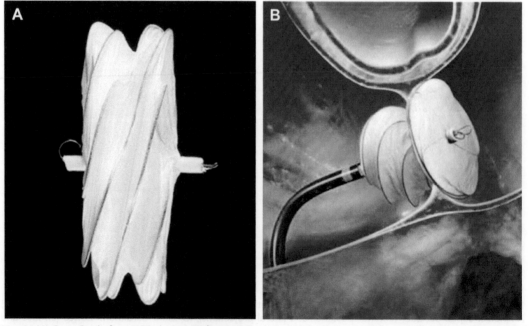

Fig. 3. (*A*) Gore Cardioform ASD device. (*B*) Cartoon depiction of the Gore Cardioform device in situ. (*Courtesy of* W.L. Gore and Associates, Flagstaff, AZ; with permission.)

research has demonstrated that the prevalence of deficient retroaortic rim is between 40% and 60% of children referred for TC-ASD[4,9,32,33] and slightly lower in adult patients.[34] A recent case-control study using data from the Erosion Board's collection and the ASO Post-Approval Study reiterated (1) that deficient retroaortic and superior vena cava rims were present in a much higher proportion of cases than control subjects, (2) ASD were larger in diameter and larger in proportion to patient weight than in control subjects, and (3) several factors suggestive of device oversizing (balloon size much larger than static defect size or device much larger than static defect size) were more common in cases and control subjects.[28] Operators are now cautious not to allow devices to indent the retroaorta or roof of the left atrium, but debate remains about "splaying" the ASO device around the aorta as shown in **Fig. 2**. There continues to be more work to identify the factors or combination of factors that identify patients where risk of TC-ASD exceeds that of O-ASD.

It is important to reiterate that the relative clinical benefit of TC-ASD to O-ASD is well established. In head-to-head comparisons, TC-ASD has consistently demonstrated equivalent efficacy with excellent safety in comparison with O-ASD[5,35,36] with the added benefit of having significantly less discomfort, superior cosmetic results, and a shorter length of stay. Reevaluating these outcomes outside of clinical trials is challenging. There are few contemporary series comparing the results of TC-ASD and O-ASD. Large multicenter series are necessary for comparisons because of systematic differences between patients undergoing O-ASD and TC-ASD and the need for statistical adjustment to account for confounding by indication. Contemporary multicenter series of TC-ASD have demonstrated the risk of in-hospital mortality is 0% to 0.015%.[4,10,37] In the same time period, data from the Society for Thoracic Surgeons Congenital Heart Surgeons database suggest that the risk of in-hospital mortality after O-ASD is between 0.3% and 0.9% even after adjusting for preoperative risk factors.[38] Even adjusting for measurable differences in case-mix, studies have consistently demonstrated that periprocedural morbidity (ie, complications) is also significantly higher after O-ASD,[39] which is also reflected in a longer length of stay and higher hospital costs following O-ASD.[39,40] Even with uncertainty regarding what the risk of "real" current risk of erosion is (which is likely a function of

patient selection and device selection), the additional risk of erosion is unlikely to overcome the relative benefits of TC-ASD over O-ASD.

However, in light of this concern it is important to determine whether concern regarding erosion is affecting practice. Analysis of clinical registry data demonstrated that patients with deficient retroaortic rim were no less likely to receive ASO devices than those with larger retroaortic rims.[4] At the same time, analysis of administrative data has allowed, for the first time, measurement of the tendency to pursue O-ASD and TC-ASD,[4] demonstrating that before 2013, the proportion of TC-ASD was increasing, but that between 2013 and 2015 this trend reversed and the proportion of O-ASD increased slightly relative to TC-ASD (**Fig. 4**). Although this trend may reflect the reasonable desire to avoid erosions, this trend in practice would potentially have risks. Although referring patients for O-ASD inevitably reduces the risk for erosion, this practice only results in a net reduction in harm to patients if the benefit exceeds the inherently higher risks of O-ASD.

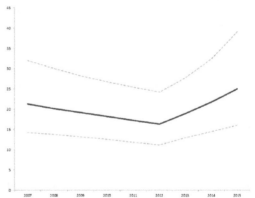

Fig. 4. Estimated probability of TC-ASD versus O-ASD 2007 to 2015. Conditional standardization was used to calculate an adjusted probability of O-ASD closure versus transcatheter device closure, for a hypothetical white six-year-old boy with no comorbid conditions (*maroon line* with 95% confidence interval represented by the dashed *gray lines*). This was based on the mixed effects multivariate generalized linear model summarized in Table 2. The probability of O-ASD closure decreased significantly from 2007 until 2012 (odds ratio, 0.95 per year; $P = .02$). In 2013, there was a significant shift in probability favoring ASD (odds ratio, 1.21 per year; $P = .006$). (*From* O'Byrne ML, Shinohara RT, Grant EK, et al. Increasing propensity to pursue operative closure of atrial septal defects following changes in the instructions for use of the Amplatzer septal occluder device an observational study using data from the pediatric health information systems database. Am Heart J 2017;192:91; with permission.)

Another trend seen in these data is a trend toward closing ASD in progressively younger patients. From the outset of TC-ASD, smaller children have had ASD closed. In the ASO device trial, there was no restriction on age or size for the TC-ASD arm, and the median age of subjects was 9.8 years with a range from 0.6 to 82 years.[5] Similarly, the first multicenter study reporting real-world use of the ASO device reporting the results of 478 cases from 13 centers performed between 2004 and 2007 demonstrated an equally broad range (infancy to the ninth decade of life).[6] In that series, 33% of reported cases were performed in patients less than 16 kg. Since that report, multiple case series demonstrate that TC-ASD can be performed even in patients less than 10 kg.[32,41–45] At the same time, most cases continue to be performed in school-age patients. Contemporary data from the IMPACT registry showed that the median age of TC-ASD is 5 to 7 years,[4,37] with a similar series from the C3PO registry reporting that 85% of subjects were older than 3 years.[10]

Although natural history studies of large ASD demonstrated a decrease in life expectancy, childhood symptoms caused by congestive heart failure were rare as was the development of pulmonary vascular disease.[46–48] Other series have demonstrated that most small defects found in infants close spontaneously.[49–51] The natural history of larger defects has not been well defined. In cross-sectional analyses, an association has been demonstrated between older patient age at diagnosis and larger defect size.[50,51] This may be caused by spontaneous closure of smaller defects, but some have hypothesized that some ASD increase in size over time.[52] This has been used as a justification for early intervention. No studies have followed ASD longitudinally to confirm if some ASD do grow over time. Even if some ASD did grow, it is unclear how often that growth would complicate TC-ASD.

Analysis of data from the PHIS registry demonstrated that the age of patients undergoing ASD closure at primary pediatric hospitals in the United States decreased progressively between 2007 and 2015,[4] independent of measurable patient-level confounders. It is impossible to determine in this study design the reasons behind this trend. Sensitivity analyses demonstrated that this was not driven by the aforementioned trend to increasing use of O-ASD and was present regardless of closure method. There is also no evidence that the trend is the result of increasing prevalence of pulmonary disease or

prematurity that might aggravate the physiologic effects of an atrial level shunt. This trend has the potential to have real ramifications on patient safety. The effect of small size on the risk of adverse events or technical failure has been equivocal in multiple studies.[4,9,10] However, McElhinney and colleagues[28] demonstrated that larger defect size to patient size was a risk factor for device erosion. Therefore, for TC-ASD, the optimal age for closure is not clear, and it remains the shared responsibility of referring physicians and interventional cardiologists to balance these risks and benefits.

These studies have demonstrated that there is more uncertainty regarding which patients should be referred for TC-ASD than what one might have expected. This is underscored by variation in the relative use of TC-ASD and O-ASD, even at large primary pediatric hospitals. Although TC-ASD accounted for greater than 80% of ASD closure procedures at US pediatric hospitals,[4] some hospitals used TC-ASD for as few as 30% of their ASD closure cases, whereas others were as high as 100%.[4] Even after adjusting for differences in case-mix, there remained significant interhospital variability in the choice between O-ASD and TC-ASD.[4] The systematic differences between hospitals underscores the lack of consensus about how ASD should be treated. Similar differences between hospitals have been seen in the distribution of indications for TC-ASD and how different hospitals define right ventricular volume overload.[53] Taken together, these observations demonstrate the lack of consensus in practice for TC-ASD and the potential benefit of standardization of practice.

MINIMALLY INVASIVE CARDIAC SURGERY

In considering the potential risk of device erosion, an important question is whether O-ASD can be made safer and less morbid for patients. Minimally invasive cardiac surgery (MICS), through "mini-sternotomy" or video-assisted thoracoscopic surgery (with or without robotic assistance), has the potential to reduce procedural morbidity relative to open heart surgery with reductions in length of stay along with improved cosmesis compared with conventional surgical correction of ASD.[54] However, to date the largest case series of MICS report lengths of stay (median, 5–7 days) that are similar to conventional studies and much longer than that following TC-ASD (1 day or less).[55–58] Enthusiasm and expertise in MICS remains limited to a few centers and is not yet a compelling alternative to conventional O-ASD and TC-ASD.

PATENT FORAMEN OVALE CLOSURE AS SECONDARY PROPHYLAXIS FOR STROKE

The incidence of cryptogenic stroke in young adults is between 15% and 35%.[59] A possible mechanism for these strokes is transient right-to-left shunt through a patent foramen ovale (PFO) allowing embolization of thrombus from the systemic venous circulation into the systemic arterial circulation (and eventually the brain). As a result, there has been significant interest in evaluating the relative benefit of device closure of PFO as secondary prophylaxis after a stroke. Three randomized clinical trials from 2012 to 2013 using the Amplatzer PFO occluder (St. Jude Medical)[60,61] and the STARFlex closure system (NMT Medical, Boston, MA)[62] failed to demonstrate benefit over medical therapy. Therefore, 2016 American Academy of Neurology recommendations stated that there was insufficient evidence to endorse device closure of PFO after cryptogenic stroke.[63] However, two recent randomized clinical trials have demonstrated a significant benefit of TC-PFO over medical therapy: the REDUCE[64] and CLOSE[65] trials. The two more recent studies differed from prior studies in that they restricted enrollment to patients in whom a right-to-left shunt could be elicited on bubble-study echocardiogram. Several meta-analyses have been applied to these data, pooling data from previous trials. The most recent of these[66] demonstrated that the benefit of device closure was greater in patients with larger right-to-left shunt (ie, a larger number of microbubbles) on agitated saline contrast echocardiogram and in the subgroup of patients less than 45 years. The pooled benefit over medical therapy was still modest (number needed to treat between 28 and 64 to prevent one stroke over 4 years depending on which estimate of stroke recurrence risk was used), but supported the benefit of TC-PFO over medical therapy.[66] Concerns over the increase in risk of atrial fibrillation with TC-PFO seem to be largely driven by events in cases where the STARFlex system was used and there was no significant difference in major adverse events between TC-PFO and medical therapy groups in this meta-analysis.[66] Additionally, reanalysis of the RESPECT trial data after longer follow-up time (median, 5.9 years, compared with previously published data after a median of 2.1 years) demonstrated significant benefit to TC-PFO over medical therapy

consistent with REDUCE and CLOSE, and demonstrating increased benefit in larger shunts on agitated saline injection.[67]

The Amplatzer PFO occluder and the Gore Cardioform device are approved by the US Food and Drug Administration for the closure of PFO as secondary prophylaxis for stroke. As these results disseminate, it is likely that pediatric/congenital cardiologists will be asked to be involved in PFO closure in adults and in children. Several questions are important to consider when translating the data from clinical trials and meta-analyses to clinical practice. First, the definition of cryptogenic stroke differs between studies and needs to be clarified to provide an accurate measurement of recurrence risk and to determine patients in whom TC-PFO closure is less likely to be effective. Second, in light of modest benefits in absolute risk reduction, it is important to determine what factors (in addition to relatively young age and larger shunt) identify populations that would benefit more from TC-PFO. Third, as with any new application of a technique there is the potential for new or unexpected adverse events along with the anticipated benefits. For example, several studies have shown that a small but significant minority of patients with ASD and PFO devices develop aortic insufficiency after device closure.[9,68–70] Addressing all of these issues requires continued vigilance and ongoing clinical effectiveness research as PFO closure becomes more widespread.

Another important issue for pediatric/congenital cardiologists is the applicability of these findings to the pediatric population. The incidence of arterial stroke is lower in children than in older patients, but the proportion of cryptogenic strokes is similar to that in adults, between 15% and 27%.[71–73] It is tempting to extrapolate data from clinical trials in older populations because the benefits TC-PFO are more robust in younger (i.e. <45 years) adults,[66,67] and because children and adolescents presumably spend more time at risk than even young adults. Documented issues with maintaining patients on chronic antiplatelet or anticoagulant regimens are likely to be even more challenging in the pediatric population. However, there is still of dearth of data in children and it is not a given that recurrence risk for cryptogenic stroke will be similar between pediatric and adult populations. In addition, to the cryptogenic stroke population an open question is whether patients' long-term central venous lines or transvenous pacing leads should be screened for PFO and which of these patients should have their PFO treated. Also, transient ischemic attacks (TIA) are a potentially problematic indication for TC-PFO. TIA are not only much more frequent than cerebrovascular accidents, but also are more problematic from a diagnostic perspective, because they are not always accompanied by findings on neuroimaging studies and have overlap in symptoms with migraines and other conditions. Diagnosis of TIA in a pediatric population is also more challenging because of the cognitive development of the population. Further research is necessary to clarify these issues and until that time, there is uncertainty regarding the appropriate care of these children.

NONIMPLANT DEFECT CLOSURE

Although most closure techniques for ASDs and PFOs rely on implantation of a permanent device within the defect, such as an Amplatzer device or Cardioform device, the ideal closure device would not use a foreign body. This "ideal" ASD closure device would obviate concern over thrombus formation, embolization, erosion, arrhythmias, and the ability to access the left atrium later in life. Clearly, with the increase in interventions for atrial fibrillation, mitral valve dysfunction, and left atrial appendage occlusion, transcatheter access to the left atrium is valuable and permanent implants in the atrial septum can make this much more difficult. Although the initial "nondevice" closure techniques have been used predominantly for closure of PFOs, it is important to consider these creative techniques because similar technology could someday be used for ASD closures.

The initial concept for nondevice closure of ASDs used radiofrequency (RF) energy to essentially "weld" together the tissue flaps or tunnel, which created a PFO. By applying RF energy to heat tissue flaps while pushing them together or using a vacuum to keep the septum primum and secundum opposed to one another, the injury and heat created from the RF energy allows the tissue to become adherent and then to heal together. The pathology of RF closure of PFOs in animals has been described and reported in a porcine model[74] and the first human implant was performed in 2005.[75] This is marketed as the RFx closure system (Cierra Inc, Redwood City, CA). In a study of 144 patients lead by Dr. Horst Sievert, the RFx device was found to be safe because there were no significant adverse

events in any of the patients except one patient who received a blood transfusion for blood loss during the procedure. However, at 6-month follow-up 45% of the PFOs continued to have a significant shunt. The device was much more effective (72% closure at 6 months) in closing smaller PFOs with stretch diameters less than 8 mm.[76]

Another new device that is being used in Europe and now also in North America is the NobleStitch device made by HeartStitch (Fountain Valley, CA). This device works by passing two sutures through different aspects of the PFO and creating a knot to suture the PFO into a closed position (**Fig. 5**). This device and its accessories are CE marked for cardiovascular suturing and PFO closure in Europe. Although this device is not approved in the United States for PFO closure, it is now being used off label for this procedure. The first reported series of cases with this device were reported in a prospective study from 12 centers in Italy.[77] This study enrolled 192 patients who were considered acceptable candidates for suture-mediated PFO closure. The NobleStitch EL system was technically successfully in 96% of the patients with no procedural or long-term complications reported. At follow-up time of about 7 months, contrast echocardiography with Valsalva showed no shunting in 75% but a "significant" shunt was seen in 11% of the patients. Although use of RF energy may be difficult to translate to significant ASD, it may be possible in the future to use a stitch-based device to close small ASD and even larger ASD with transcatheter patch placement in the future. It may also become possible to use these sorts of techniques along with device closure to minimize the risks of either erosion or embolization for high-risk ASDs.

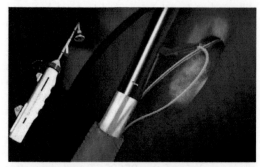

Fig. 5. NobleStitch EL device for PFO closure. (*Left*) NobleStitch EL device. (*Right*) Drawing of mechanism of action of the device demonstrating mechanism of action of stitch placement. (*Courtesy of* HeartStitch® Inc. [Fountain Valley, CA].)

SUMMARY

Transcatheter device closure of defects in the interatrial septum have been performed for more than 40 years and have demonstrated excellent safety and efficacy. The controversy surrounding the risk of device erosion has brought to light the lack of consensus among different centers as to how to approach this lesion. Continued innovation in development of devices and epidemiologic surveillance of practice are necessary to provide the best care for patients with ASD.

REFERENCES

1. Hoffman JIE, Kaplan S. The incidence of congenital heart disease. J Am Coll Cardiol 2002;39:1890–900.
2. King TD, Thompson SL, Steiner C, et al. Secundum atrial septal defect. Nonoperative closure during cardiac catheterization. JAMA 1976;235:2506–9.
3. King TD, Mills NL. Historical perspective on ASD device closure. In: Hijazib ZM, Feldman T, Abdullah Al-Qbandi MH, Sievert H, editors. Transcatheter closure of ASDs and PFOs. Minneapolis (MN): Cardiotext; 2010. p. 37–64.
4. O'Byrne ML, Gillespie MJ, Kennedy KF, et al. The influence of deficient retro-aortic rim on technical success and early adverse events following device closure of secundum atrial septal defects: an analysis of the IMPACT Registry(®). Catheter Cardiovasc Interv 2017;89:102–11.
5. Du ZD, Hijazi ZM, Kleinman CS, et al, Amplatzer Investigators. Comparison between transcatheter and surgical closure of secundum atrial septal defect in children and adults: results of a multicenter nonrandomized trial. J Am Coll Cardiol 2002;39:1836–44.
6. Everett AD, Jennings J, Sibinga E, et al. Community use of the Amplatzer atrial septal defect occluder: results of the multicenter MAGIC atrial septal defect study. Pediatr Cardiol 2008;30:240–7.
7. Wang J-K, Tsai S-K, Wu M-H, et al. Short- and intermediate-term results of transcatheter closure of atrial septal defect with the Amplatzer septal occluder. Am Heart J 2004;148:511–7.
8. Knepp MD, Rocchini AP, Lloyd TR, et al. Long-term follow up of secundum atrial septal defect closure with the Amplatzer septal occluder. Congenit Heart Dis 2010;5:32–7.
9. O'Byrne ML, Glatz AC, Sunderji S, et al. Prevalence of deficient retro-aortic rim and its effects on outcomes in device closure of atrial septal defects. Pediatr Cardiol 2014;35:1181–90.
10. El-Said H, Hegde S, Foerster S, et al. Device therapy for atrial septal defects in a multicenter cohort: acute outcomes and adverse events. Catheter Cardiovasc Interv 2015;85:227–33.
11. Vincent RN, Raviele AA, Diehl HJ. Single-center experience with the HELEX septal occluder for closure of atrial septal defects in children. J Interv Cardiol 2003;16:79–82.
12. Jones TK, Latson LA, Zahn E, et al. Results of the U.S. multicenter pivotal study of the HELEX septal occluder for percutaneous closure of secundum atrial septal defects. J Am Coll Cardiol 2007;49:2215–21.
13. Latson LA, Jones TK, Jacobson J, et al. Analysis of factors related to successful transcatheter closure of secundum atrial septal defects using the HELEX septal occluder. Am Heart J 2006;151:1129.e7-11.
14. Correa R, Zahn E, Khan D. Mid-term outcomes of the Helex septal occluder for percutaneous closure of secundum atrial septal defects. Congenit Heart Dis 2013;8:428–33.
15. de Hemptinne Q, Horlick EM, Osten MD, et al. Initial clinical experience with the GORE(®) Cardioform ASD occluder for transcatheter atrial septal defect closure. Catheter Cardiovasc Interv 2017. https://doi.org/10.1002/ccd.26907.
16. Preventza O, Sampath-Kumar S, Wasnick J, et al. Late cardiac perforation following transcatheter atrial septal defect closure. Ann Thorac Surg 2004;77:1435–7.
17. Chun DS, Turrentine MW, Moustapha A, et al. Development of aorta-to-right atrial fistula following closure of secundum atrial septal defect using the Amplatzer septal occluder. Catheter Cardiovasc Interv 2003;58:246–51.
18. Trepels T, Zeplin H, Sievert H, et al. Cardiac perforation following transcatheter PFO closure. Catheter Cardiovasc Interv 2003;58:111–3.
19. Amin Z, Hijazi ZM, Bass JL, et al. Erosion of Amplatzer septal occluder device after closure of secundum atrial septal defects: review of registry of complications and recommendations to minimize future risk. Catheter Cardiovasc Interv 2004;63:496–502.
20. Amplatzer septal occluder and delivery system: instructions for use. 2012. Available at: professional.sjm.com. Accessed November 25, 2013.
21. United States Food and Drug Administration. Rare serious erosion events associated with St. Jude Amplatzer atrial septal occluder (ASO). Silver Spring (MD): United States Food and Drug Administration; 2013.
22. Mallula K, Amin Z. Recent changes in instructions for use for the Amplatzer atrial septal defect occluder: how to incorporate these changes while using transesophageal echocardiography or intracardiac echocardiography? Pediatr Cardiol 2012;33:995–1000.
23. DiBardino DJ, McElhinney DB, Kaza AK, et al. Analysis of the US Food and Drug Administration

Manufacturer and User Facility Device Experience database for adverse events involving Amplatzer septal occluder devices and comparison with the Society of Thoracic Surgery congenital cardiac surgery database. J Thorac Cardiovasc Surg 2009;137: 1334–41.

24. Delaney JW, Li JS, Rhodes JF. Major complications associated with transcatheter atrial septal occluder implantation: a review of the medical literature and the manufacturer and user facility device experience (MAUDE) database. Congenit Heart Dis 2007;2:1–9.

25. DiBardino DJ, Mayer JE Jr. Continued controversy regarding adverse events after Amplatzer septal device closure: mass hysteria or tip of the iceberg? J Thorac Cardiovasc Surg 2011;142:222–3.

26. Diab K, Kenny D, Hijazi ZM. Erosions, erosions, and erosions! Device closure of atrial septal defects: how safe is safe? Catheter Cardiovasc Interv 2012; 80:168–74.

27. Moore J, Hegde S, El-Said H, et al. Transcatheter device closure of atrial septal defects: a safety review. JACC Cardiovasc Interv 2013;6:433–42.

28. McElhinney DB, Quartermain MD, Kenny D, et al. Relative risk factors for cardiac erosion following transcatheter closure of atrial septal defects: a case-control study. Circulation 2016; 133:1738–46.

29. Taggart NW, Dearani JA, Hagler DJ. Late erosion of an Amplatzer septal occluder device 6 years after placement. J Thorac Cardiovasc Surg 2011;142: 221–2.

30. Roberts WT, Parmar J, Rajathurai T. Very late erosion of Amplatzer septal occluder device presenting as pericardial pain and effusion 8 years after placement. Catheter Cardiovasc Interv 2013; 82:E592–4.

31. Amin Z. Echocardiographic predictors of cardiac erosion after Amplatzer septal occluder placement. Catheter Cardiovasc Interv 2014;83:84–92.

32. Petit CJ, Justino H, Pignatelli RH, et al. Percutaneous atrial septal defect closure in infants and toddlers: predictors of success. Pediatr Cardiol 2012;34:220–5.

33. O'Byrne ML, Glatz AC, Goldberg DJ, et al. Accuracy of transthoracic echocardiography in assessing retro-aortic rim prior to device closure of atrial septal defects. Congenit Heart Dis 2014. https:// doi.org/10.1111/chd.12226.

34. Butera G, Romagnoli E, Carminati M, et al. Treatment of isolated secundum atrial septal defects: impact of age and defect morphology in 1,013 consecutive patients. Am Heart J 2008;156:706–12.

35. Kutty S, Abu Hazeem A, Brown K, et al. Long-term (5- to 20-year) outcomes after transcatheter or surgical treatment of hemodynamically significant isolated secundum atrial septal defect. Am J Cardiol 2012;109:1348–52.

36. Kotowycz MA, Therrien J, Ionescu-Ittu R, et al. Long-term outcomes after surgical versus transcatheter closure of atrial septal defects in adults. JACC Cardiovasc Interv 2013;6:497–503.

37. Moore JW, Vincent RN, Beekman RH, et al. Procedural results and safety of common interventional procedures in congenital heart disease: initial report from the National Cardiovascular Data Registry. J Am Coll Cardiol 2014;64:2439–51.

38. O'Brien SM, Clarke DR, Jacobs JP, et al. An empirically based tool for analyzing mortality associated with congenital heart surgery. J Thorac Cardiovasc Surg 2009;138:1139–53.

39. Ooi YK, Kelleman M, Ehrlich A, et al. Transcatheter versus surgical closure of atrial septal defects in children: a value comparison. JACC Cardiovasc Interv 2016;9:79–86.

40. O'Byrne ML, Gillespie MJ, Shinohara RT, et al. Cost comparison of transcatheter and operative closures of ostium secundum atrial septal defects. Am Heart J 2015;169:727–35.e2.

41. Wyss Y, Quandt D, Weber R, et al. Interventional closure of secundum type atrial septal defects in infants less than 10 kilograms: indications and procedural outcome. J Interv Cardiol 2016;29:646–53.

42. Abu-Tair T, Wiethoff CM, Kehr J, et al. Transcatheter closure of atrial septal defects using the GORE® septal occluder in children less than 10 kg of body weight. Pediatr Cardiol 2016;37:778–83.

43. Tanghöj G, Odermarsky M, Naumburg E, et al. Early complications after percutaneous closure of atrial septal defect in infants with procedural weight less than 15 kg. Pediatr Cardiol 2016;38: 255–63.

44. Fischer G, Smevik B, Kramer HH, et al. Catheter-based closure of atrial septal defects in the oval fossa with the Amplatzer® device in patients in their first or second year of life. Catheter Cardiovasc Interv 2009;73:949–55.

45. Fraisse A, Losay J, Bourlon F, et al. Efficiency of transcatheter closure of atrial septal defects in small and symptomatic children. Cardiol Young 2008;18:343–7.

46. Campbel M. Natural history of atrial septal defect. Br Heart J 1970;32:820–6.

47. Craig RJ, Selzer A. Natural history and prognosis of atrial septal defect. Circulation 1968;37:805–15.

48. Andersen M, Lyngborg K, Moller I, et al. The natural history of small atrial septal defects: long-term follow-up with serial heart catheterizations. Am Heart J 1976;92:302–7.

49. Radzik D, Davignon A, van Doesburg N, et al. Predictive factors for spontaneous closure of atrial septal defects diagnosed in the first 3 months of life. J Am Coll Cardiol 1993;22:851–3.

50. Hanslik A, Pospisil U, Salzer-Muhar U, et al. Predictors of spontaneous closure of isolated secundum

atrial septal defect in children: a longitudinal study. Pediatrics 2006;118:1560–5.

51. Helgason H, Jonsdottir G. Spontaneous closure of atrial septal defects. Pediatr Cardiol 1999;20:195–9.

52. McMahon CJ, Feltes TF, Fraley JK, et al. Natural history of growth of secundum atrial septal defects and implications for transcatheter closure. Heart 2002;87:256–9.

53. O'Byrne ML, Kennedy KF, Rome JJ, et al. Variation in practice patterns in device closure of atrial septal defects and patent ductus arteriosus: an analysis of data from the IMproving Pediatric and Adult Congenital Treatment (IMPACT) registry. Am Heart J 2018;196:119–30.

54. Bacha E, Kalfa D. Minimally invasive paediatric cardiac surgery. Nat Rev Cardiol 2014;11:24–34.

55. Lee H, Yang J-H, Jun T-G, et al. The mid-term results of thoracoscopic closure of atrial septal defects. Korean Circ J 2017;47:769–75.

56. Burkhart HM, Suri RM. Minimally invasive video assisted surgical closure of secundum atrial septal defect. Ann Cardiothorac Surg 2017;6:60–3.

57. Kodaira M, Kawamura A, Okamoto K, et al. Comparison of clinical outcomes after transcatheter vs. minimally invasive cardiac surgery closure for atrial septal defect. Circ J 2017;81:543–51.

58. Schneeberger Y, Schaefer A, Conradi L, et al. Minimally invasive endoscopic surgery versus catheter-based device occlusion for atrial septal defects in adults: reconsideration of the standard of care. Interact Cardiovasc Thorac Surg 2016. https://doi.org/10.1093/icvts/ivw366.

59. Ferro JM, Massaro AR, Mas J-L. Aetiological diagnosis of ischaemic stroke in young adults. Lancet Neurol 2010;9:1085–96.

60. Carroll JD, Saver JL, Thaler DE, et al. Closure of patent foramen ovale versus medical therapy after cryptogenic stroke. N Engl J Med 2013;368:1092–100.

61. Meier B, Kalesan B, Mattle HP, et al. Percutaneous closure of patent foramen ovale in cryptogenic embolism. N Engl J Med 2013;368:1083–91.

62. Furlan AJ, Reisman M, Massaro J, et al. Closure or medical therapy for cryptogenic stroke with patent foramen ovale. J Med 2012;366:991–9.

63. Messé SR, Gronseth G, Kent DM, et al. Practice advisory: recurrent stroke with patent foramen ovale (update of practice parameter): report of the guideline development, dissemination, and implementation Subcommittee of the American Academy of Neurology. Neurology 2016;87:815–21.

64. Sondergaard L, Kasner SE, Rhodes JF, et al. Patent foramen ovale closure or antiplatelet therapy for cryptogenic stroke. N Engl J Med 2017;377:1033–42.

65. Mas J-L, Derumeaux G, Guillon B, et al. Patent foramen ovale closure or anticoagulation vs. antiplatelets after stroke. N Engl J Med 2017;377:1011–21.

66. Akobeng AK, Abdelgadir I, Boudjemline Y, et al. Patent foramen ovale (PFO) closure versus medical therapy for prevention of recurrent stroke in patients with prior cryptogenic stroke: a systematic review and meta-analysis of randomized controlled trials. Catheter Cardiovasc Interv 2018;92:165–73.

67. Saver JL, Carroll JD, Thaler DE, et al. Long-term outcomes of patent foramen ovale closure or medical therapy after stroke. N Engl J Med 2017;377:1022–32.

68. Schoen SP, Boscheri A, Lange SA, et al. Incidence of aortic valve regurgitation and outcome after percutaneous closure of atrial septal defects and patent foramen ovale. Heart 2008;94:844–7.

69. Wöhrle J, Kochs M, Spiess J, et al. Impact of percutaneous device implantation for closure of patent foramen ovale on valve insufficiencies. Circulation 2009;119:3002–8.

70. Loar RW, Johnson JN, Cabalka AK, et al. Effect of percutaneous atrial septal defect and patent foramen ovale device closure on degree of aortic regurgitation. Catheter Cardiovasc Interv 2013;81:1234–7.

71. Mackay MT, Wiznitzer M, Benedict SL, et al, International Pediatric Stroke Study Group. Arterial ischemic stroke risk factors: the international pediatric stroke study. Ann Neurol 2011;69:130–40.

72. Mallick AA, Ganesan V, Kirkham FJ, et al. Childhood arterial ischaemic stroke incidence, presenting features, and risk factors: a prospective population-based study. Lancet Neurol 2014;13:35–43.

73. Gerstl L, Weinberger R, Kries von R, et al. Risk factors in childhood arterial ischaemic stroke: findings from a population-based study in Germany. Eur J Paediatr Neurol 2018;22:380–6.

74. Hara H, Jones TK, Ladich ER, et al. Patent foramen ovale closure by radiofrequency thermal coaptation: first experience in the porcine model and healing mechanisms over time. Circulation 2007;116:648–53.

75. Sievert H, Fischer E, Heinisch C, et al. Transcatheter closure of patent foramen ovale without an implant: initial clinical experience. Circulation 2007;116:1701–6.

76. Sievert H, Ruygrok P, Salkeld M, et al. Transcatheter closure of patent foramen ovale with radiofrequency: acute and intermediate term results in 144 patients. Catheter Cardiovasc Interv 2009;73(3):368–73.

77. Gaspardone A, De Marco F, Sgueglia GA, et al. Novel percutaneous suture-mediated patent foramen ovale closure technique: early results of the NobleStitch EL Italian Registry. EuroIntervention 2018;14:e272–9.

New Patent Ductus Arteriosus Closure Devices and Techniques

Hitesh Agrawal, MD[a], Benjamin Rush Waller III, MD[a],
Sushitha Surendan, MD[b], Shyam Sathanandam, MD[b],*

KEYWORDS

- PDA • Premature • MVP • AVP II • ADO II AS

KEY POINTS

- Patent ductus arteriosus (PDA) in extremely low-birth-weight infants should be evaluated and managed by a multidisciplinary team, including neonatologists, cardiac surgeons, and cardiologists.
- Transcatheter PDA occlusion is a viable and safe procedure for hemodynamically significant PDAs even in small, preterm infants and can lead to better outcomes.
- These procedures should be limited to specialized centers with expertise in these transcatheter procedures.

INTRODUCTION

Patent ductus arteriosus (PDA) is very common in preterm neonates and can be found in ~42% of infants weighing less than 1200 g.[1–3] The PDAs in this group of neonates are relatively larger, more distensible, and longer than PDAs in older children and are referred to as "fetal type or type F PDAs."[4] The presence of PDA puts them at increased risk of chronic lung diseases, necrotizing enterocolitis, intraventricular hemorrhage, longer hospitalization, and higher mortality.[5] Hemodynamically significant PDA is defined based on clinical and transthoracic echocardiographic (TTE) evaluation. Such patients commonly have respiratory failure requiring mechanical ventilation. Important echocardiographic (ECHO) features include size ≥2 mm, left heart enlargement, and pan-diastolic flow reversal in the abdominal aorta.

A multidisciplinary team approach is required for the management of PDAs in preterm neonates. Medical therapy is not very effective, and surgical ligation, although can be performed in all cases, poses undue risks, including bleeding, pneumothorax, phrenic nerve palsy, vocal cord paralysis, and chylous effusion.[6–8]

Transcatheter closure of PDA is considered standard of care in patients weighing greater than 5 kg. However, with the advancement in transcatheter devices, it can now be performed safely in extremely low-birth-weight (ELBW) neonates with low risk of complications.[9,10] In this article, the authors describe approaches and techniques for transcatheter closure of PDA in ELBW preterm infants.

PATIENT SELECTION

To allow for input from multiple teams with a variety of expertise, patients should be discussed in a multidisciplinary team meeting comprising of the patient's neonatologists, cardiac surgeons, and cardiologists. All hemodynamically significant PDAs would qualify for transcatheter closure except those with active infection, hemodynamic or respiratory instability that precludes

[a] Pediatric Interventional Cardiology, University of Tennessee, LeBonheur Children's Hospital, 848 Adams Avenue, Memphis, TN 38103, USA; [b] Department of Pediatric Interventional Cardiology, University of Tennessee, LeBonheur Children's Hospital, 848 Adams Avenue, Memphis, TN 38103, USA
* Corresponding author.
E-mail address: shyam@uthsc.edu

Intervent Cardiol Clin 8 (2019) 23–32
https://doi.org/10.1016/j.iccl.2018.08.004
2211-7458/19/© 2018 Elsevier Inc. All rights reserved.

transfer to the catheterization laboratory, intracardiac thrombus, or severe renal dysfunction, and those with continuous right-to-left shunting across the PDA.

PREPROCEDURAL PREPARATION

PDA closure in preterm infants can be performed at bedside with ECHO and portable fluoroscopic guidance but typically is performed in the cardiac catheterization laboratory under general anesthesia using biplane fluoroscopy with the lowest frame rate of 3 frames per second. The patient is transported from the neonatal intensive care unit to the cardiac catheterization laboratory in the incubator, using either a transport ventilator or bag ventilation via an endotracheal tube. The patient is kept warm using heat lamps and a heating blanket with continuous temperature monitoring via an esophageal probe. The blood pressure (BP) cuff is placed around the left lower extremity and is cycled every 5 minutes. TTE is performed by the operator standing at the head side of the table, and a note is made in regards to the ideal windows for scanning during the procedure. Baseline measurements of the PDA diameters at the pulmonary and aortic end, and length of PDA are recorded. The systolic pulmonary artery (PA) pressure is estimated using peak systolic gradient across the PDA and subtracting it from the systolic blood pressure. A complete hemodynamic catheterization is not performed unless there is concern for pulmonary hypertension. Typically, pulmonary hypertension does not develop until the second or third months of life. Therefore, earlier PDA closure may be beneficial for these ELBW infants.

TECHNIQUE FOR PROCEDURE

A 4-French 7-cm introducer sheath is placed in the right femoral vein under ultrasound guidance. Arterial access is not obtained because this group of patients are at high risk of arterial injury.[11] Heparinized saline flushes are sufficient to maintain activated clotting times between 200 and 250 seconds. Hence, heparin bolus is not given. Prophylactic antibiotics are administered. Under fluoroscopic guidance, a 4-French angled glide catheter (Terumo, Japan) and a 0.035″ Wholey wire (Medtronic, Minneapolis, MN, USA) are used to cross the PDA antegrade into the descending aorta. The wire is removed, and a hand injection is performed using this catheter to delineate the size of the PDA. This angiogram is performed at 15 frames per second for accurate measurements, and the largest dimensions are used for device selection.

DEVICE SELECTION

Currently approved devices for PDA occlusion in the United States (Fig. 1), such as the Amplatzer Duct Occluder (ADO; Abbott, Lake Bluff, IL, USA) and the Nitocclud (PFM Medical AG, Cologne, Germany) devices, are typically suited for conical shaped PDAs (type A morphology) that are typically encountered in older children. The PDA morphology in ELBW infants is similar to the fetal ductus arteriosus (type F morphology). The Amplatzer Duct Occluder–II (ADO-II) can be useful, but requires a relatively bulky delivery system. Coils can be delivered for PDA occlusion through small catheters. However, the PDA is such a high flow lesion that the coils can easily embolize to nontarget structures. In this section, the use of 3 devices that are currently not Food and Drug Administration approved for the closure of PDA in the ELBW infants are discussed. The devices that the authors commonly use for PDA closure in patients less than 2 kg are the microvascular plug (MVP; Medtronic), the Amplatzer ductal occluder II additional sizes (ADO II AS; Abbott, Lake Bluff, IL,

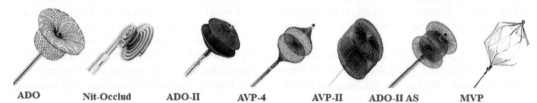

ADO   Nit-Occlud   ADO-II   AVP-4   AVP-II   ADO-II AS   MVP

Fig. 1. Some of the commercially available devices used for PDA occlusions: the ADO and the ADO-II devices are currently approved in the United States for use in children over 6 months of age and greater than 6 kg. The Nit-Occlud PDA device is approved for children greater than 5 kg. The Amplatzer vascular plug 4, AVP-4, and the AVP-II are common plugs used off label for PDA occlusions in children born prematurely. They are best suited for those greater than 2 kg. The ADO-IIAS and the MVP are perhaps good devices for PDA occlusions even for those less than 1 kg. There is an ongoing clinical trial in the United States to evaluate the safety and effectiveness of the ADO-IIAS device for PDA closure. (Courtesy of Abbott, Lake Bluff, IL, with permission; and pfm Medical ag, Cologne, Germany, with permission; and Medtronic, Minneapolis, MN, with permission.)

USA), and Amplatzer vascular plug II (AVP II, Abbott).

Microvascular Plug

The MVP is composed of a nitinol framework covered partially by a polytetrafluoroethylene (PTFE) membrane at the proximal portion. Oversizing of the device to the target vessel anchors it in place, and the PTFE covering leads to faster occlusion. The delivery wire is a 0.018″ nitinol pusher that is 180 cm long up to the detachment zone. There is a proximal and distal radiopaque marker. Mainly, 2 sizes of the device are used in premature neonates: 5.3 mm (MVP-3Q) and 6.5 mm (MVP-5Q), which can be introduced through microcatheters of inner diameters of 0.021″ and 0.027″, respectively. The unconstrained length is 12 mm for both sizes, whereas the maximal constrained length is 15 and 16 mm for the MVP-3Q and MVP-5Q, respectively. The MVP-3Q is recommended for target vessel diameter between 1.5 and 3 mm and the MVP-5Q for 3- to 5-mm diameter PDA. The MVP-7Q is 9-mm unconstrained diameter and can be used for larger PDAs between 5- and 7-mm diameter via a 4-French catheter.

The device comes in a dispenser tube attached to a delivery wire. The device is prepared by immersing it into heparinized saline and withdrawing it into the loader catheter by pulling the delivery wire until the tip of the MVP is sheathed. The distal end of the introducer sheath is inserted into the hub of the 4-French glide catheter that has already been placed in the PDA through a Y-connector. After flushing the system, the hemostasis valve is tightened. The pusher wire is then advanced through the 4-French angle glide catheter until the distal platinum marker of the MVP is aligned with the distal part of the catheter. The hemostasis valve is then loosened, and the device is unsheathed by slowly pulling back on the glide catheter while maintaining a constant forward pressure on the delivery wire. An angiogram is performed through the Y-adapter connected to the end of the glide catheter in a caudal angulation on the frontal and straight lateral projections to rule out any stenosis of the left pulmonary artery (LPA). TTE is used to delineate any residual shunting or obstruction to the descending aorta or to the LPA (Fig. 2). If repositioning of MVP is desired, the 4-French glide catheter is readvanced over the delivery wire to recapture the device, and the device can be redeployed in the same manner. Once satisfactory position is achieved, the device can be detached using a torque device.

Although the MVP can be delivered through a microcatheter, the 4-French glide catheter is preferable, because it allows for an angiogram to be performed if necessary as well as to recapture the device before release or even after releasing the device using a snare. The MVP is not a very radiopaque device (Fig. 3). Having the distal radiopaque marker to match the esophageal temperature probe on lateral fluoroscopy is a good technique to avoid excessive protrusion of the device into the aorta. Cycling of the BP cuff in the lower extremity as well as palpation of the femoral arterial pressure can confirm good aortic flow. TTE can be used for confirmation. An angiogram performed via the Y-connector can help confirm that the device does not obstruct the PAs. The MVP is a fairly long device. MVP is advantageous to cover the entire PDA length. The PDA is quite long in the ELBW infant. The smaller the patient, the longer the PDA.[12] Therefore, this device is best suited for the tiniest of patients.

In the authors' series, they have performed PDA occlusions successfully on 72 ELBW infants between 600 g and 1500 g, with one failed attempt. The failure was secondary to the device not implanted properly. The device had displaced more proximal than expected causing mild LPA stenosis. Although this 700-g patient was hemodynamically stable, the authors elected to retrieve the device. A 5-mm snare was used to capture the proximal radiopaque pin, and the device was sheathed entirely into the 4-French glide catheter and retrieved without any complication. The PDA was occluded using an ADO-II AS device. There was one 900-g patient with a residual shunt noted on the postprocedure TTE following the implantation of an MVP-7Q plug in a 6-mm PDA. The shunt was not visualized on follow-up TTE. The residual shunting was attributed to a small tear in the Gore-Tex membrane, which can happen due to repeated recapture and repositioning of the device. It is recommended that a new device be used after more than 3 attempts to reposition the MVP.

Because the MVP does not have any retention discs, it avoids obstruction of the LPA or the aorta and may be more suited in the extremely small-sized patients. Oversizing the device by 1 to 2 mm greater than the PDA will eliminate the potential risk of embolization. In a series of 146 ELBW infants with PDA closure at less than less than 2 kg from the authors' institution, the median diameter of the PDA was 3.5 mm at the PA end, 4.2 mm at the aortic end, and 10.6 mm in length based on angiographic

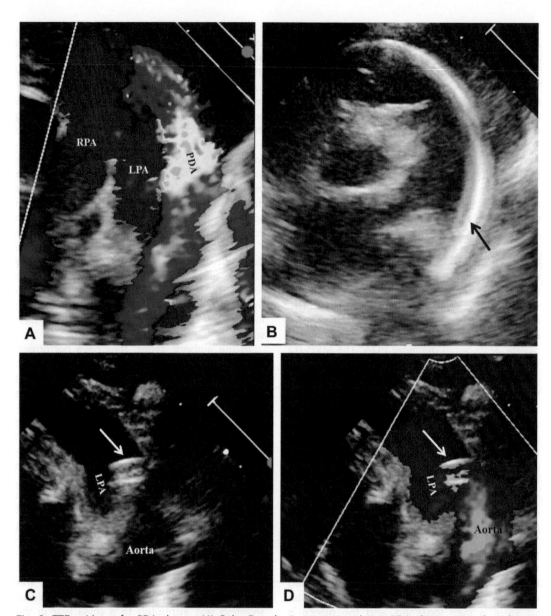

Fig. 2. TTE guidance for PDA closure. (*A*) Color Doppler interrogation during PDA closure procedure demonstrating a large PDA with left-to-right shunting in a 24 weeks' gestation ELBW infant, who is now 2 weeks old and weighs 700 g. RPA, right pulmonary artery. (*B*) Parasternal short-axis view demonstrating a catheter (*arrow*) being advanced through the right ventricular outflow tract into the PDA. (*C, D*) Two-dimensional (2D)-TTE with color Doppler interrogation after device deployment (*arrows*) within the PDA demonstrating no stenosis of the LPA or the aorta.

measurement. Therefore, the MVP-5Q is almost a one-size-fits-all for patients of this size. These extremely small patients do not tolerate stiff wires across the tricuspid and pulmonary valves that are required to advance a delivery sheath for device deployment. The delivery cable of the MVP is less stiff compared with other devices, and consequentially, easier to maneuver through the heart in neonates weighing as small as 600 g. The MVP also has the advantage of being delivered through the same catheter that is used to cross the PDA, avoiding the need for a sheath exchange. There have been no other adverse events with the use of the MVP. In the authors' series, the procedure and fluoroscopic times while using the MVP for PDA occlusions are a median of 24 (range 8–44) and 4 (range 1.4–7.8) minutes, respectively.

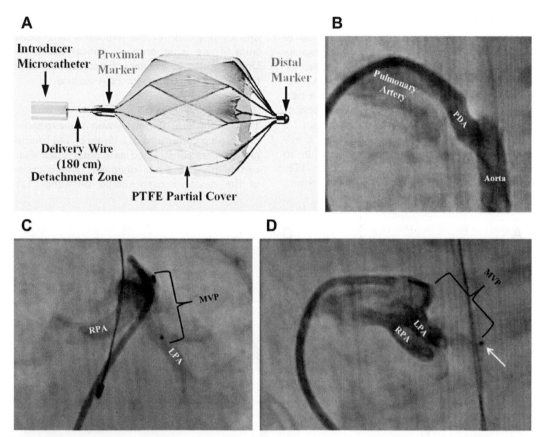

Fig. 3. PDA closure using the MVP in a 24-weeks' gestation infant, who is 3 weeks of age and weighs 900 g. (*A*) The MVP with the parts labeled. (*B*) Angiogram in a straight lateral projection to demonstrate a large type F PDA before device closure. (*C*) Angiogram performed in the PA after PDA occlusion using the MVP in a caudal angulation demonstrating no stenosis of the branch pulmonary arteries. (*D*) Same angiogram viewed in a straight lateral projection demonstrating no stenosis of the branch pulmonary arteries. The arrow points to the distal radiopaque marker lined up to the temperature probe in the esophagus. (*Courtesy of* Medtronic, Minneapolis, MN; with permission.)

Amplatzer Duct Occluder II Additional Sizes

The ADO II AS is a self-expanding occlusion device with a central waist and retention disc on both ends designed to minimize the protrusion into the aortic and PA. The retention discs on either side are 1 to 1.5 mm greater than the central device. The sizes are based on the central device and are available in 3 sizes. Therefore, the 3-mm device has discs 4 mm in size; the 4-mm device has discs that are 5.25 mm in size, and the 5-mm device has 6.5-mm disc sizes. It can be used for PDAs ≤4 mm in diameter and at least 3 mm in length. It can be placed through a 4-French delivery catheter via the venous approach in this population. Therefore, a catheter exchange is needed. The authors recommend using the 0.035″ Wholey wire for catheter exchange. In general, this wire is very atraumatic and is likely to not injure any valve structures or the PDA, unlike lower-caliber wires.

Also, using a 0.035″ wire reduces wire catheter mismatch, preventing any adverse event due to that. The central waist fills up the ductal lumen, and the retention discs are designed to deploy in the pulmonary and the aortic end of the ductus arteriosus. However, in ELBW infants, the authors recommend delivering the entire device intraductally, preventing any chance of inadvertent stenosis to the distal aortic arch or the LPA. Hence, ADO II AS allows for relative undersizing of the device because it allows for the sizing to be based on the retention disc size rather than the central device. Although these PDAs are long, the authors recommend the use of the 2-mm-length device. Again, the length of the device is only that of the central waist and not that of the entire device. The unconstrained length of the 2-mm device is actually 6 mm, and it can lengthen up to 10 mm. Therefore, the 4-2 ADO-II AS could again be a one-size-fits-all PDAs in ELBW infants. It comes pre-attached to a delivery cable, the distal tip of which is extremely flexible and is angiographically visible, which helps in precise placement of the device within the ductus (**Fig. 4**). After device placement, a PA angiography can be performed through the Y-connector at the end of the delivery catheter. The aortic end can be checked using the principles described previously, including lining up the distal marker to the esophageal temperature probe, TTE, lower-extremity noninvasive BP measurement before and after device occlusion of the PDA, and by palpation of the femoral arterial pulsations. There is an ongoing clinical trial in the United States to evaluate the safety and effectiveness of this device for PDA closure.

Amplatzer Vascular Plug II

The AVP II is a densely woven self-expanding nitinol plug composed of 2 layers of 144 braided nitinol wires constructed as 2 outer discs and a central plug of equal diameter. The diameter of the device chosen should be either 1 to

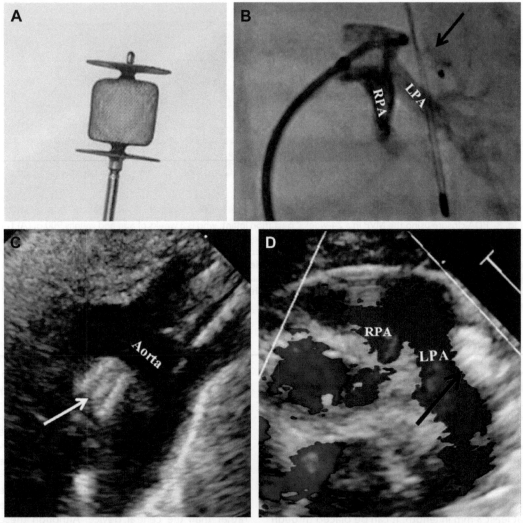

Fig. 4. PDA closure using the ADO-IIAS in a 23-weeks' gestation infant, who is 3 weeks of age and weighs 760 g. (A) The ADO-IIAS device. Note how the retention discs on either side is larger than the central portion. (B) Angiogram in a straight lateral projection after device occlusion demonstrating no obstruction to either branch pulmonary arteries. The arrow points to the device still attached to the delivery cable. Device can be retrieved or repositioned if the positioning is found not to be ideal. (C) 2D-TTE demonstrating the ADO-IIAS device (*arrow*) to be completely intraductal with no obstruction to the aorta. (D) Color Doppler interrogation of the PA demonstrating no LPA stenosis. Note the TEE demonstrating the ADO-IIAS device (*arrow*) still attached to the delivery cable. (*Courtesy of* Abbott, Lake Bluff, IL; with permission.)

2 mm larger or 20% larger than the target vessel. It can accomplish rapid PDA occlusion. The 4-mm and the 6-mm AVP-II can be delivered using a long 4-French sheath. It has excellent fluoroscopic and ECHO visibility (Fig. 5).

The PDA is crossed as described above. Over a 0.025″ wire parked in the descending aorta via the PDA, a 4-French hydrophilic sheath (Flexor; Cook Medical, Bloomington, IN, USA) is advanced into the descending aorta. An appropriate sized AVP-II is prepared and loaded into the introducer delivery catheter by pulling back on the delivery wire under heparinized saline. The device introducer is inserted into the long delivery sheath, and the AVP-II is advanced to the tip of the sheath in the descending aorta. Once appropriate position of the device is achieved in the PDA, it is unsheathed while exerting mild forward tension on the device to maintain it within the ductus arteriosus. If the device position is suboptimal, it can be recaptured by advancing the 4-French sheath over the delivery wire. Once satisfactory position is achieved, the device is detached from the delivery wire followed by an angiogram and removal of the sheath.

The disadvantages of the AVP-II include the need for a sheath exchange, relatively stiff delivery cable, and unavailability of a 5-mm device. Above features make this device not ideal for very small infants. Although the authors have used this device frequently in the past, more recently they have only used the AVP-II for PDA occlusions in children greater than 2 kg. Of the 117 PDA occlusions performed using the AVP-II at the authors' center, only 22 were performed in children less than 2 kg, and only 3 were performed in children under 1 kg. In contrast, all 72 MVP used for PDA occlusions were performed in children less than 1.5 kg, with 38 occlusions in children less than

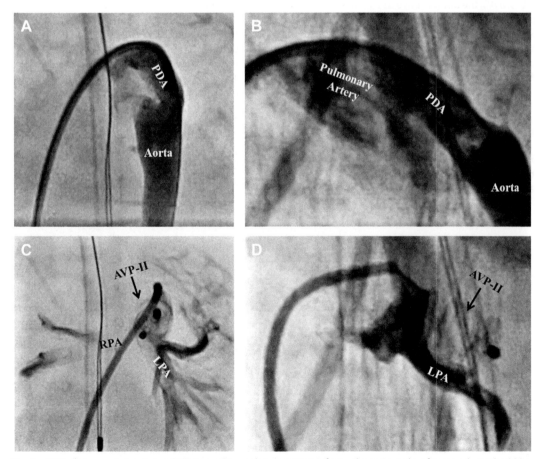

Fig. 5. PDA closure using a 6-mm AVP-II in a 24-weeks' gestation infant, who is 4 weeks of age and weighs 980 g. (*A*, *B*) Straight AP and lateral projection of an angiogram performed via an antegrade catheter in the PDA demonstrating a large PDA in this ELBW infant. (*C*, *D*) Straight AP and lateral projection of an angiogram performed via an antegrade catheter in the PA demonstrating adequate intraductal positioning of the device with no stenosis of the branch pulmonary arteries. (*Courtesy of* Abbott, Lake Bluff, IL; with permission.)

1 kg. The AVP-II was successful in 94% of the times when attempted. There was a 5% incidence of LPA stenosis with the AVP-II exclusively when used in children less than 1.2 kg (Fig. 6), although retrieval of the AVP-II was necessary in only 2 patients in whom the device was successfully snared and sheathed into a long 4-French sheath. In both these patients (900 g and 1100 g in weight, respectively), the PDA went into spasm after retrieval and did not require further intervention. There was one device embolization in a 3-kg infant noted 4 hours after device implant that was successfully retrieved. The patient underwent surgical ligation of the PDA.

One of the other limitations is the unavailability of a 5-mm AVP-II. In children less than 2 kg, the PDA is typically around 3 to 4 mm, which likely requires a 5-mm device. The authors have had several instances in which the 4-mm AVP-II was too small and the 6-mm AVP-II was too big. More recently, with the availability of the MVP and the ADO-II AS, the authors have used the AVP-II in children greater than 2 kg only. The stiff delivery cable keeps the tricuspid valve in an open position, thereby limiting cardiac output during device implantation, which occurs least with the use of the MVP compared with other devices.

TIPS AND TRICKS FOR PATENT DUCTUS ARTERIOSUS DEVICE OCCLUSION IN EXTREMELY LOW-BIRTH-WEIGHT INFANTS

From operators experienced with the occlusion of hundreds of PDAs in premature infants, these are a few of the lessons that have been learned:

1. ELBW infants are very sensitive to rapid hemodynamic and thermodynamic changes and must be handled with extreme caution.
2. Only femoral venous access should be obtained in ELBW infants. Arterial access can lead to complications.
3. Ultrasound should be used to prevent inadvertent femoral arterial injury during femoral venous access.
4. Catheter and wire manipulation in these children must be gentle and purposeful.
5. Adverse events can be mitigated with a graded decrease in the patient size, until a level of comfort performing transcatheter PDA closure in ELBW infants smaller than 1 kg can be achieved.
6. Heparin bolus administration should be avoided in ELBW infants. Heparinized flushes can be used to prevent thrombosis within catheters.
7. The 4-French, 65-cm angled glide catheter (Terumo) and the 0.035″ Wholey wire (Medtronic) are the best catheter and wire to use for ELBW infants. Avoiding wire-catheter mismatch is important to prevent vessel injury and to the tricuspid valve.
8. The PDA in ELBW infant is long and tubular, resembling the fetal ductus, and typically 4 mm in diameter and 10 mm in length. Therefore, the MVP-5Q and the 4-2 ADO-II AS are basically one-size-fits-all PDAs in ELBW infants.
9. Device should be implanted entirely intraductal to prevent inadvertent stenosis

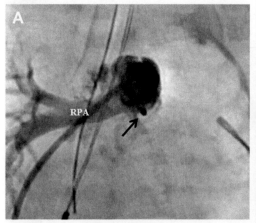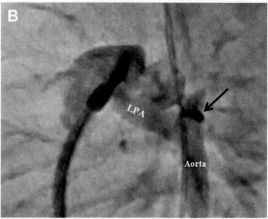

Fig. 6. Complications of PDA closure using the AVP-II. (A) Angiogram performed using an antegrade catheter in the PA after PDA closure using a 6-mm AVP-II in a 24-weeks' gestation ELBW infant weighing 1000 g during the procedure. Note the complete occlusion of the left PA by the device (arrow). The device was retrieved using a 5-mm snare into a 4-French Mullin sheath. The PDA went into spasm and never reopened. (B). Angiogram performed through the delivery sheath with a 6-mm AVP-II device still attached to the delivery cable in this 1080-g ELBW infant. The arrow points to the distal disc causing obstruction of the descending aorta. The device was retrieved, and the PDA was closed using an MVP-5Q device. (Courtesy of Abbott, Lake Bluff, IL; with permission.)

of the LPA or the distal aortic arch. Discless devices such as the MVP can prevent this complication.

10. Stiff delivery cables and catheters keep the tricuspid valve open and lead to decreased cardiac output during device delivery. Therefore, the MVP and the ADO-II AS are ideally suited for children less than 2 kg.
11. Real-time TTE can be used to determine ideal device positioning. TTE guidance eliminates the need for arterial access and aortograms.
12. TTE tends to underestimate the PDA length. The smaller the patient, the longer the PDA. As the child gets older, the PDA tends to shorten.
13. A hand injection of contrast can be used to determine ideal device positioning in the pulmonary end and to rule out LPA stenosis.
14. Useful techniques to check ideal device positioning at the aortic end and to rule out distal aortic arch obstruction include the use of TTE and Doppler interrogation, lining up the distal marker of the device to a previously placed esophageal temperature probe, lower-extremity noninvasive BP measurement before and after device occlusion of the PDA, and by palpation of the femoral arterial pulsations.
15. Ideal timing for PDA closure in ELBW infants is within the first 4 week of age beyond which the benefit is limited. By 8 weeks, most ELBW infants with a large PDA show evidence of pulmonary hypertension.
16. Clinically apparent postligation syndrome seen with surgical PDA ligation is not encountered with device occlusion in ELBW infants.

FOLLOW-UP CARE

All premature infants who undergo PDA device closure should undergo clinical evaluation, including an ECHO and chest radiograph, 6-hours after the procedure. It was routine to perform surveillance ultrasound and venous Doppler interrogation 1 week after transcatheter PDA occlusion only for infants 2 kg; but as no complications were noted in the authors' series, this practice was abandoned after the initial few. A cardiac clinical examination is performed once a week until hospital discharge. ECHO evaluation is performed 30 days after closure. The authors have instituted a multidisciplinary PDA clinic for longer-term follow-ups. All these patients are followed in the PDA clinic for a period of 3 years to assess for any longer-term issues, including pulmonary and neurodevelopmental outcomes.

DISCUSSION

Transcatheter closure of PDA in ELBW neonates represents a paradigm shift that has come about from collaboration between the neonatologists, cardiologists, pulmonologists, and cardiac surgeons. There are a multitude of factors that determine the feasibility and success of a program planning to undertake such procedures. It cannot be overemphasized that these ELBW neonates are extremely vulnerable and cannot tolerate any complications. There is a learning curve to this procedure, and small details matter. Important predictors include early referral for the procedure, experience in transporting these neonates to and from the catheterization laboratory, precise and accurate measurements, and speedy performance of the procedure. As in any other areas of medicine, the success of a program depends also on support from institutional leadership. Equipment manufacturers need to be involved to create and miniaturize catheters and devices. It is very important that these patients who undergo this procedure are followed carefully, so that long-term safety, benefits to patients, and outcomes can be clearly studied.

SUMMARY

Hemodynamically significant PDAs in preterm neonates can cause significant morbidity and mortality. A multidisciplinary team approach is required in the evaluation and management for optimal outcome. A repertoire of PDA occlusion devices are now available that can be safely used to close PDAs in extremely small neonates. The techniques described above represent the authors' institutional experience and has helped us to streamline the procedure.

REFERENCES

1. Dice JE, Bhatia J. Patent ductus arteriosus: an overview. J Pediatr Pharmacol Ther 2007;12(3):138–46.
2. Ellison RC, Peckham GJ, Lang P, et al. Evaluation of the preterm infant for patent ductus arteriosus. Pediatrics 1983;71(3):364–72.
3. Hammerman C. Patent ductus arteriosus. Clinical relevance of prostaglandins and prostaglandin inhibitors in PDA pathophysiology and treatment. Clin Perinatol 1995;22(2):457–79.
4. Philip R, Waller BR, Agrawal V, et al. Morphologic characterization of the patent ductus arteriosus in the premature infant and the choice of transcatheter occlusion device. Catheter Cardiovasc Interv 2016;87(2):310–7.

5. Jim W-T, Chiu N-C, Chen M-R, et al. Cerebral he-modynamic change and intraventricular hemor-rhage in very low birth weight infants with patent ductus arteriosus. Ultrasound Med Biol 2005;31(2): 197–202.

6. Koehne PS, Bein G, Alexi-Meskhishvili V, et al. Pat-ent ductus arteriosus in very low birthweight infants: complications of pharmacological and surgical treatment. J Perinat Med 2001;29(4):327–34.

7. Zbar RIS, Chen AH, Behrendt DM, et al. Incidence of vocal fold paralysis in infants undergoing ligation of patent ductus arteriosus. Ann Thorac Surg 1996; 61(3):814–6.

8. Seghaye MC, Grabitz RG, Alzen G, et al. Thoracic sequelae after surgical closure of the patent ductus arteriosus in premature infants. Acta Paediatr 1997; 86(2):213–6.

9. Zahn EM, Peck D, Phillips A, et al. Transcatheter closure of patent ductus arteriosus in extremely premature newborns: early results and midterm follow-up. JACC Cardiovasc Interv 2016;9(23): 2429–37.

10. Sathanandam S, Justino H, Waller BR, et al. Initial clinical experience with the Medtronic Micro Vascular Plug™ in transcatheter occlusion of PDAs in extremely premature infants. Catheter Cardio-vasc Interv 2017;89(6):1051–8.

11. Alexander J, Yohannan T, Abutineh I, et al. Ultra-sound-guided femoral arterial access in pediatric cardiac catheterizations: a prospective evaluation of the prevalence, risk factors, and mechanism for acute loss of arterial pulse. Catheter Cardiovasc Interv 2016;88(7):1098–107.

12. Paudel G, Philip R, Zurakowski D, et al. Echocardio-graphic guidance for trans-catheter device closure of patent ductus arteriosus in extremely low birth weight infants. JACC 2018;71(11 Supplement). https://doi.org/10.1016/S0735-1097(18)31117-3.

Pulmonary Artery Stenting

Jenny E. Zablah, MD*, Gareth J. Morgan, MB, BaO, BCh

KEYWORDS

- Pulmonary artery stenosis • Stent placement • Catheter intervention • Congenital heart disease

KEY POINTS

- Pulmonary artery stenosis is heterogenous, with a wide morphology in multiple forms of congenital heart disease and genetic syndromes.
- Primary intravascular stent implantation is recommended in significant branch pulmonary artery stenosis when the vessel or patient is large enough to accommodate a stent that can be dilated to an adult diameter.
- A variety of specialized stents are now available, improving applicability despite complex vessel size characteristics; however, developments in bioresorbable stents and patient-specific rapid prototyping are anticipated.

INTRODUCTION

Pulmonary artery disease can include stenotic or hypoplastic vessels, and those compressed by other structures, such as the aorta or bronchi. The pathologic conditions are heterogenous throughout multiple forms of congenital heart disease and genetic syndromes. Stent implantation is a branch of treatment options that also include balloon angioplasty and surgical augmentation.

INDICATIONS FOR INTERVENTION

There are several indications for intervention (balloon angioplasty and/or stent implantation) on the pulmonary arteries but, usually, these relate to objective measurements of decreased flow to the affected lung and/or a significant pressure gradient across the area of stenosis, which may result in increases in right ventricular pressure.[1] Current recommendations for primary intravascular stent implantation include significant branch pulmonary artery stenosis when the vessel or patient is large enough to accommodate a stent capable of being dilated to an adult diameter of the vessel.

Despite the recommendations and common practice, it is also reasonable to implant small pulmonary artery stents that lack the potential to achieve adult size in small children as part of a strategy to palliate significant branch pulmonary artery stenosis in special situations. This should be evaluated on a case by case basis. Newer stent designs combine lower delivery profiles for use in smaller patients with either improved redilation potential or the possibility to fracture the stent if needed as the vessel grows.

THE LIMITATIONS OF ANGIOPLASTY

Studies of acute and intermediate-term success results showed that balloon angioplasty of pulmonary arteries is statistically less effective than stent placement.[2] Currently, the role of balloon dilation is somewhat limited. Balloon angioplasty alone is indicated for severe pulmonary artery stenosis, particularly in very small patients or in those in whom stent implantation is not a viable option due to complex anatomy. Although angioplasty is relatively easy to perform and needs small vascular access, if it is performed with balloons only slightly larger in

The authors do not have a financial interest in or arrangement or affiliation with any organization that could be perceived as a real or apparent conflict or interest in the context of the subject of this publication.

Department of Pediatric Cardiology, Children's Hospital of Colorado, University of Colorado School of Medicine, 13123 East 16th Avenue, Box 100, Aurora CO 80045, USA

* Corresponding author.

E-mail address: jenny.zablah@childrenscolorado.org

diameter than the treated vessel, the stenosis might be dilated but without permanent results. When considerably larger balloons are used, the chance of effective reduction of the obstruction is higher but the rate of complications increases, including vessel rupture or dissection. It is important to also consider that if the pulmonary artery is being externally compressed by other structures, balloon angioplasty will not be effective because the cause of the obstruction is secondary to mechanical compression instead of primary vessel abnormality.

STENT IMPLANTATION

Pulmonary artery stents are indicated in main or branch pulmonary artery stenosis that is not expected to have an adequate response to primary pulmonary artery balloon dilation. Stents are effective for congenital pulmonary artery stenosis, postsurgical stenosis, or stenosis due to external compression by other structures.

Types of Stents–Advantages and Disadvantages
Open-cell or hybrid design versus closed-cell stents
Open-cell stents have 2 major advantages: they usually have a larger final diameter and they allow dilation through its side cells into the orifice of potential jailed side branches (Table 1). On the other hand, closed-cell stents are easier to crimp onto a balloon and they have intrinsically higher radial strength (Fig. 1).

Unmounted versus premounted stents
Unmounted stents can usually reach larger diameters but must be mounted onto a balloon with length that matches as closely as possible the length of the stent. The premounted stents, in contrast, are small to medium diameter, need smaller delivery systems (6–7F), and have better trackability and flexibility. For these reasons, they are advantageous in infants and small children.

Balloon expanded versus self-expanding stents
Self-expanding stents are highly flexible but with less predictable deployment when compared with balloon-expandable stents. They cannot be easily dilated beyond their nominal diameter. Balloon-expandable stents, on the other hand, have increased radial strength with predictable placement but have less flexibility (Fig. 2).

Covered versus bare-metal stents
Covered stents are especially useful in very narrow stenotic vessels because they provide an additional seal to avoid vessel dissection and bleeding in extremely stressed vessels. Covered stents are also useful to cover and isolate areas of dissection or aneurysm. The disadvantages of this type of stent include the necessity for larger sheaths to accommodate the covering and the difficulty encountered when a covered stent is deployed in a position where an important side branch is crossed. Bare-metal stents are far more widely used in the pulmonary arteries for all these and other reasons (Fig. 3).

TECHNIQUES
Percutaneous
Although there are variations between experienced operators' practices, and newer techniques and indications call for an open-minded approach to deployment, the standard and safe approach toward pulmonary artery stent deployment can be concisely described. After hemodynamic and angiographic assessment with exact measurements of the target lesion and the upstream and downstream vasculature, a distal guide wire position must be achieved. A long sheath advanced over the wire is positioned into the pulmonary artery to facilitate stent placement. The catheter with the mounted stent is advanced over the guidewire and through the long sheath to sit astride the lesion. The stent is uncovered and small-volume hand-injected angiography can be performed through the sheath to confirm and optimize positioning. For balloon-expandable stents (by far the most commonly used in the pulmonary arteries), the sheath is then withdrawn to a safe distance proximal to the balloon before inflating the balloon to expand the stent against the vessel wall. The balloon is then fully deflated and carefully removed, leaving the wire in place and the sheath nearby to facilitate repeat diagnostics or other interventions. Following deployment of the stent, hemodynamic and angiographic assessment is performed.

Hybrid Intraoperative Stent Placement
This approach can be useful in smaller patients and in patients with complex anatomy in whom placing a stent in the catheterization laboratory may be too difficult, or percutaneous stent placement may interfere with concurrent or subsequent operations. Such procedures are performed jointly by cardiac surgeons and interventional cardiologists. The exact conduct of these procedures is variable. It may encompass a minimal

Table 1
Types of stents and characteristics

Stent	Premounted	Covered	Balloon vs Self-Expandable	Cell Design	Available Diameters (mm)	Available Lengths (mm)	Sheath Size Required (F)
Atrium iCAST Atrium Medical Corporation, Hudson, NH, USA	Yes	Yes	Balloon-expandable	Closed	5–10	16–59	6–7
Cordis PALMAZ Blue Cordis Fremont, CA, USA	Yes	No	Balloon-expandable	Closed	4–7	12–24	4–5
Cordis PALMAZ Genesis Cordis Fremont, CA, USA	Yes	No	Balloon-expandable	Closed	3–10	12–80	5–8
BARD Valeo BARD Peripheral Vascular, Inc, Temple, AZ, USA	Yes	No	Balloon-expandable	Open	6–10	18–56	6–7
Cook Medical Formula 418 Cook Medical, Bloomington, IN, USA	Yes	No	Balloon-expandable	Open	3–8	12–30	5–8
Boston Scientific VeriFLEX Boston Scientific, Marlborough, MA, USA	Yes	No	Balloon-expandable	Open	2.75–5	8–32	5–6
Abbott Omnilink Elite Abbott Laboratories, Abbott Park, IL, USA	Yes	No	Balloon-expandable	Open	6–10	12–59	6–7
RX Herculink Elite Renal Stent System Abbott Laboratories, Abbott Park, IL, USA	Yes	No	Balloon-expandable	Open	4–7	12–18	6
Cordis PALMAZ Genesis XD Cordis Fremont, CA, USA	No	No	Balloon-expandable	Closed	10–18	19–59	8
Bare CP Stent 8 zig NuMED Inc, NY, USA	No	No	Balloon-expandable	Closed	12–24	16–60	10–12
Bare CP Stent 10 zig NuMED Inc, NY, USA	No	No	Balloon-expandable	Closed	26–30	39–60	16

(continued on next page)

Stent	Premounted	Covered	Balloon vs Self-Expandable	Cell Design	Available Diameters (mm)	Available Lengths (mm)	Sheath Size Required (F)
Covered Mounted CP Stent NuMED Inc, NY, USA	Yes	Yes	Balloon-expandable	Closed	12–30	16–60	12–18
Cordis PALMAZ XL Cordis Fremont, CA, USA	No	No	Balloon-expandable	Closed	14–25	30–50	12–14
IntraStent Max LD Medtronic, MN, USA	No	No	Balloon-expandable	Open	12	16–36	11
IntraStent Mega LD Medtronic, MN	No	No	Balloon-expandable	Open	9–12	16–36	9
IntraStent DoubleStrut LD Medtronic, MN, USA	No	No	Balloon-expandable	Open	5–18	16–76	8
AndraStent XL and XXL Andramed GmbH, Reutlingen, Germany	No	No	Balloon-expandable	Hybrid	15–32	13–57	7–11
Dynalink Biliary stent Abbott Laboratories, Abbott Park, IL, USA	Yes	No	Self-expandable	Hybrid	5–10	28–100	6
Protégé GPS Medtronic, MN, USA	Yes	No	Self-expandable	Hybrid	6–14	20–80	6
Cook Zilver Cook Medical, Bloomington, IN, USA	Yes	No	Self-expandable	Hybrid	6–10	20–80	7

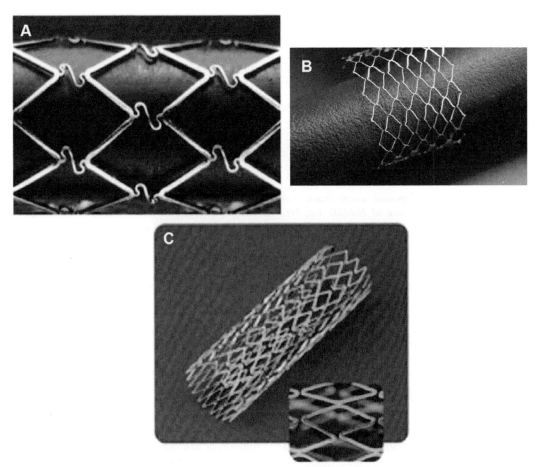

Fig. 1. (*A*) PALMAZGenesis (closed-cell). (*B*) AndraStent (hybrid). (*C*) IntraStent Max LD (open-cell). (*Courtesy of* [A] Cordis, Inc, Fremont, CA, USA, with permission; and [B] Andramed GmbH, Reutlingen, Germany, with permission; and [C] Medtronic, Minneapolis, MN, USA, with permission.)

thoracotomy or ministernotomy with a purse-string placed to allow convenient sheath placement, followed by fluoroscopic and angiographically guided stent placement, through to procedures performed on full cardiopulmonary bypass and circulatory arrest. In those cases, the surgeon provides direct access to the abnormal segment of pulmonary artery, allowing sheath, then stent, placement under direct visualization.

OUTCOMES
Short-Term
Branch pulmonary artery stenting can be considered successful if there is improvement of the right ventricular pressures and of the pulmonary artery size, or with improvement of the gradient across the target lesion of greater than 50%. The overall procedural success for procedures in biventricular hearts has been reported to

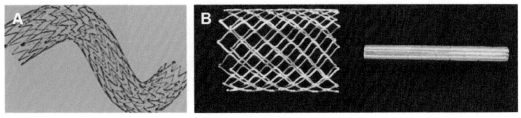

Fig. 2. (*A*) Self expanding stent (Innova). (*B*) Balloon-expandable stent (IntraStent DoubleStrut LD). (*Courtesy of* [A] Boston Scientific, Marlborough, MA, USA, with permission; and [B] Medtronic, Inc, Minneapolis, MN, USA, with permission.)

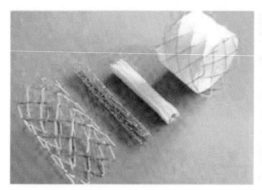

Fig. 3. Bare-metal and covered stents (bare and covered CP Stent). (*Courtesy of* NuMED Inc, NY, USA; with permission.)

be 76% (95% confidence interval [CI] 73%–79%) and patients with a single ventricle had a successful intervention in 75% (95% CI 70%–80%) of cases.[3]

In isolated discrete stenosis, stent implantation can result in complete relief of the obstruction, resulting in decrease in pressure gradients to a normalization of right ventricular pressures and improvement of flow distribution to the branch pulmonary arteries. The immediate expected outcome is angiographic improvement of the pulmonary artery diameter with improved distal flow (Fig. 4).

In multiple stenosis, an attempt to treat the most severe and proximal stenosis is an adequate approach and, in many situations, a single stent can relieve multiple areas of concern. The overall result in these cases with many sites of stenosis are variable and it may

take serial cardiac catheterizations to reach the expected result.

Medium to Long-Term

Neointimal proliferation normally covers the inner surface of the stent within 6 months after implantation. When there is a great degree of neointimal proliferation, it may cause restenosis of the vessel. The rate of restenosis has been reported between 1.5% and 4%[4] (Fig. 5).

Redilation of the stents is commonly required due to neointimal proliferation, somatic growth of the patient, or elective expansion through serial dilation to avoid overdilation.

POSTPROCEDURAL CARE

After effective treatment of the pulmonary artery stenosis with a stent, placement is important to monitor respiratory status, especially in patients with high pulmonary artery pressures with improved severe pulmonary stenosis because of possible reperfusion injury.

Owing to implantation of the stent, prophylactic antibiotic coverage is indicated based on each center's protocol after foreign body implantation.

In many centers, anticoagulation with 24-hour heparin or low-dose aspirin is performed, especially if a small diameter stent is placed, because of increased risk of thrombus formation before epithelialization.

Serial follow-up with echocardiography is useful to anticipate when further intervention, including stent redilation, is indicated based on increased gradients across the stent.

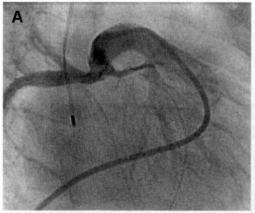
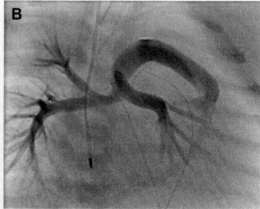

Fig. 4. Angiographic improvement of left pulmonary artery (LPA) stenosis in a patient with hypoplastic left heart syndrome status post Norwood procedure and Sano shunt. Baseline angiogram (*A*) showed long segment of LPA stenosis with significant improvement after stent placement (*B*).

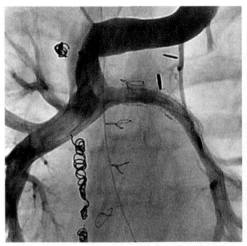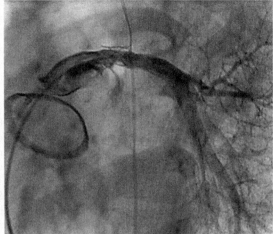

Fig. 5. Intimal growth is seen within the stents of these patients.

COMPLICATIONS

In a multicenter study with data obtained from the National Cardiovascular Data Registry–IMPACT Registry, 14% (95% CI 12%–16%) of all procedures of pulmonary artery stenting involved a complication and 9% (95% CI 7–11) of all procedures had a major adverse event. Weight less than 4 kg, emergency procedures, and single ventricle status were significantly associated with the risk of any adverse event.

Vessel Rupture
Vessel rupture can cause bleeding into the interstitial lung tissue, into the airway (ie, bronchi), and into pleural space, and it can be life-threatening. If possible, the damaged vessel should be obstructed with a low-pressure balloon. It is also important to reverse anticoagulation, have blood products available for volume replacement, and to have positive-pressure ventilation.

Balloon Rupture Before Full Stent Expansion
Balloon rupture may occur in a calcified homograft, during placement of a stent within other stents, if a balloon with thin material is being used, or if difficult positioning requires a lot of manipulation. The balloon must be exchanged for another to proceed to successful deployment.

Stent Embolization
Stent embolization can be caused by undersizing the target vessel or by underestimating the compliance of the stenotic vessel. Also, it can result from stent misplacement. If the stent has moved into a reachable area, an attempt can be made to introduce a slightly larger balloon and load the stent on it by careful inflation and repositioning after capturing on the balloon. Snare removal may also be attempted. The final resort is surgical removal.

NEW AND UPCOMING TECHNOLOGY
Bioresorbable Stents
There has been a focus on bioresorbable scaffold technologies as the next step in stent evolution. Despite a lack of evidence-based data in coronary artery trials, the industry and investigators remain hopeful that this branch of technology will play a future role. Such technology is particularly exciting for pediatric use. It may allow stent placement in small children without limiting future vessel growth because of complete resorption of any foreign material from the wall of the pulmonary artery.

Rapid Prototyping
The rapid prototyping technique quickly fabricates a scale model of a stent using 3-dimensional (3D) computer-aided design data. Construction of the stent for a specific patient anatomy would be possible with 3D printing or so-called additive layer manufacturing technology. This will allow personalized stents to be made that will target specific lesions in patients with complex cardiac anatomy.

Modifiable or Breakable Stents
Although in congenital cardiology it has become customary to break the struts of stents that were not designed to facilitate this, some investigators have moved toward manufacturing stents that break automatically after a time or allow easy disruption of key portions of their structure.

These can be implanted in infants and small children, allowing dilation to adult size without mechanical restrictions. One such stent is the Growth Stent, QualiMed (Winsen [Luhe], Germany). This stent is made of 2 separate longitudinal halves of laser-cut and electropolished 0.16-mm stainless steel. The halves are connected by a series of polydioxanone bioabsorbable sutures, which loses half of its strength within 5 weeks of implantation and is completely absorbed after about 6 months[5] (Fig. 6).

SPECIFIC LESIONS

Pulmonary artery stenosis is a very heterogenous lesion and can be characterized by the patient's anatomy or other comorbidities.

Discrete Stenosis

Discrete branch pulmonary artery stenosis it is most commonly due to anastomotic scars after congenital patchplasty, reanastomosis, or other procedures that include the pulmonary arteries, such as systemic to pulmonary artery shunts, Glenn anastomosis, and Fontan procedures (Fig. 7).

Long-Segment Stenosis

Long-segment stenosis of the branch pulmonary arteries is rarely responsive to balloon angioplasty alone and stenting is almost always the choice to relieve the obstruction (Fig. 8).

Bilateral Proximal Pulmonary Artery Stenosis

Bilateral pulmonary artery stenosis involving the ostia of the branches may require special techniques to avoid each stent compromising the contralateral vessel or the contralateral stent. These lesions can be technically challenging. Simultaneous deployment of the stents in each branch can be performed; however, this usually requires 2 large caliber long sheaths to be in place at the same time (Fig. 9). Alternatively, a long hybrid or open-cell stent can be placed, intentionally jailing the origin of the contralateral stent. Following this, the other branch of the pulmonary artery is accessed through the struts of the first stent and another stent placed through this area. The technique in which a Y-shaped stent complex is created is probably better tolerated, more predictable, and more reliable than simultaneous stent deployment (Fig. 10).

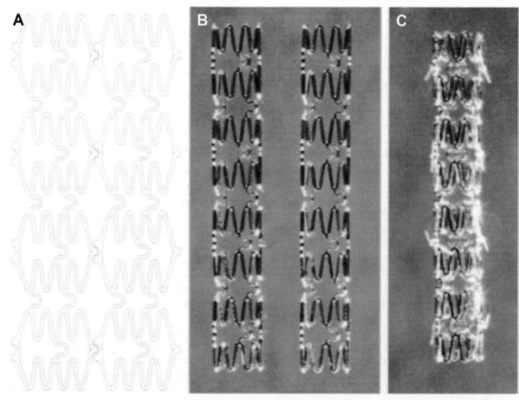

Fig. 6. (A) Drawing of the Growth Stent. (B) Picture of the stent divided in half. (C) Finished stent with the bioabsorbable sutures in place.

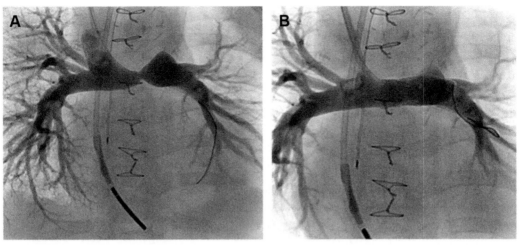

Fig. 7. (A) Proximal LPA discrete stenosis in a patient with bidirectional Glenn anastomosis. (B) The same patient after stent placement in the LPA with angiographic improvement.

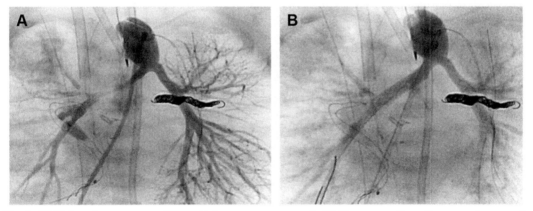

Fig. 8. (A) Right pulmonary artery (RPA) with long-segment stenosis. (B) The same patient after stent placement in the RPA.

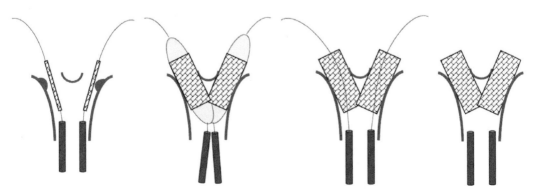

Fig. 9. Technique of simultaneous deployment of stents in each branch pulmonary artery.

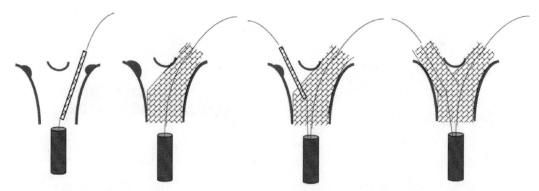

Fig. 10. Technique of Y-shaped stent complex is created to relief proximal bilateral pulmonary artery stenosis.

Distal Branch Pulmonary Artery Stenosis

Multilobar and subsegmental stenoses are frequently associated with Williams and Alagille syndromes. Often, these branches are hypoplastic down to the distal pulmonary vasculature (Fig. 11). Usually, serial balloon angioplasty is needed to rehabilitate these pulmonary arteries because stent placement has the risk of jailing off multiple small branches. There are situations in which balloon angioplasty is not effective, then placement of an open-cell stent is an option for better result, and it is always possible to open its side cells to maintain patency of flow to small branches.[6]

External Compression Pulmonary Artery Stenosis

External compression is a relatively common cause of proximal branch pulmonary artery stenosis in congenital heart disease. The right pulmonary artery is more often compressed because it runs below the aortic arch, between the ascending and descending aorta. Bilateral pulmonary artery stenosis is usually seen after the Lecompte maneuver in patients with transposition of great arteries. This is a result of the stretching of the branch pulmonary arteries when moved anteriorly to the right ventricle, resulting in straddling of the ascending aorta. External compression stenosis almost always requires stent placement to have an adequate relief of the obstruction[7] (Figs. 12 and 13).

SPECIFIC RELATED CONGENITAL HEART DISEASE OR GENETIC SYNDROMES
Williams Syndrome

Branch pulmonary artery stenosis is the second most common cardiovascular abnormality in

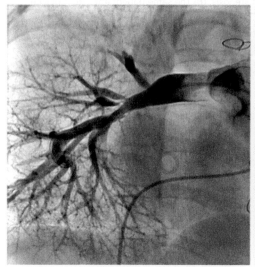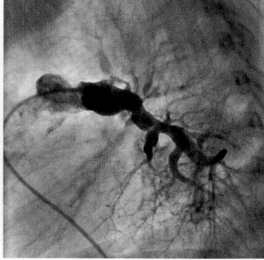

Fig. 11. Hypoplastic distal pulmonary vasculature in a patient with Alagille syndrome.

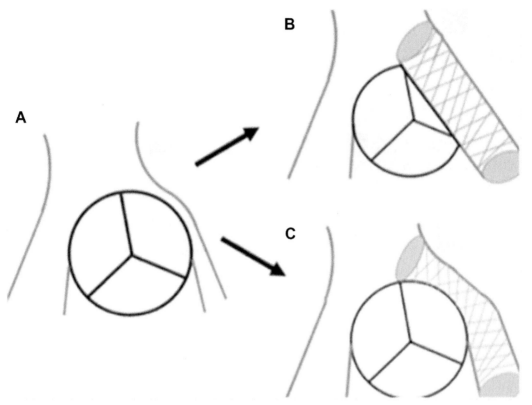

Fig. 12. Potential interaction between the aorta and the pulmonary artery (A) using a balloon-expandable stent (B) and a self-expanding stent (C) in a stretched LPA after Lecompte maneuver.

this population. The stenosis most commonly occurs in the branch and peripheral pulmonary arteries. These are diffuse stenoses involving large segments of the pulmonary arterial tree. The natural history is improvement with time; therefore intervention might be indicated based on the severity of the lesions[8] (Fig. 14).

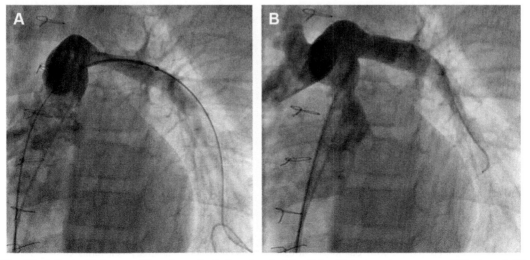

Fig. 13. Patient with transposition of great arteries s/p arterial switch with Lecompte maneuver. LPA stenosis (A) was treated with a self-expanding stent (B) with a good angiographic result.

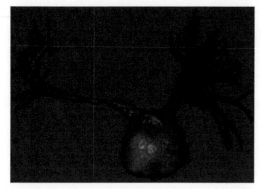

Fig. 14. 3D rotational angiography reconstruction in a patient with William syndrome and RPA diffuse stenosis.

Multiple Aortopulmonary Collaterals

After unifocalization, multiple aortopulmonary collaterals are attached to the native vessels and are very high risk for restenosis. Also, these vessels have an abnormal structure and usually have sharp angles with difficult access[9] (Fig. 15).

Pulmonary Artery Aneurysm in Pulmonary Hypertension

Patients with pulmonary hypertension may develop aneurysm in the affected pulmonary artery branches with high risk of rupture. In these cases, isolation of the affected branch can be an alternative to surgery. This is possible using a covered stent that will maintain patency of the main branch pulmonary artery and stop flow to the aneurysmal branch (Fig. 16).

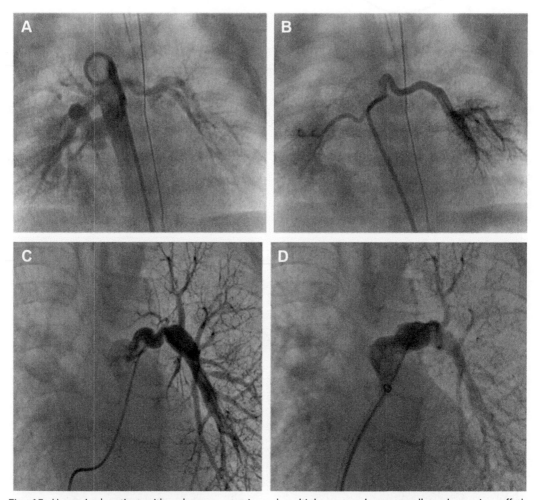

Fig. 15. Unrepaired patient with pulmonary atresia and multiple aortopulmonary collaterals coming off the descending aorta (A, B). Patient s/p unifocalization of multiple aortopulmonary collaterals with tortuous neo-LPA (C) with improved angiographic appearance after stent placement (D).

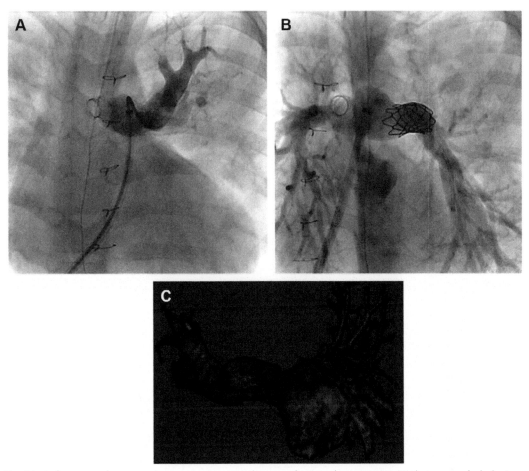

Fig. 16. Left upper pulmonary artery aneurysm secondary to pulmonary hypertension (A) that was excluded using a covered CP Stent in the proximal LPA (B). A 3D rotational angiography reconstruction of an RPA aneurysm seen in a different patient (C).

SUMMARY

Stent implantation for pulmonary artery stenosis has come far, driven by technological developments alongside innovative and ground-breaking thinking by investigators. Newer generations of stents allow confidence in long-term results, even when intervening in infants and small children. Developments in bioresorbable stents and patient-specific rapid prototyping that will open more options for complex patients with congenital heart disease are anticipated.

REFERENCES

1. Warnes CA, Williams RG, Bashore TM, et al. ACC/ AHA 2008 guidelines for the management of adults with congenital heart disease: a report of the American College of Cardiology/American Heart Association Task Force on Practice Guidelines (Writing Committee to Develop Guidelines on the Management of Adults With Congenital Heart Disease). Developed in collaboration with the American Society of Echocardiography, Heart Rhythm Society, International Society for Adult Congenital Heart Disease, Society for Cardiovascular Angiography and Interventions, and Society of Thoracic Surgeons. J Am Coll Cardiol 2008;52(23):e143–263.

2. Trant CA, O'Laughlin MP, Ungerleider RM, et al. Cost-effectiveness analysis of stents, balloon angioplasty, and surgery for the treatment of branch pulmonary artery stenosis. Pediatr Cardiol 1997;18: 339.

3. Lewis MJ, Kennedy KF, Ginns J, et al. Procedural success and adverse events in pulmonary artery stenting: insights from the NCDR. J Am Coll Cardiol 2016;67(11):13271335.

4. Shaffer KM, Mullins CE, Grifka RG, et al. Intravascular stents in congenital heart disease: short- and long-term results from a large single-center experience. J Am Coll Cardiol 1998;31(3):661–7.

5. Ewert P, Riesenkampff E, Neuss M, et al. Novel growth stent for the permanent treatment of vessel stenosis in growing children: an experimental study. Catheter Cardiovasc Interv 2004;62:506–10.

6. Trivedi KR, Benson LN. Interventional strategies in the management of peripheral pulmonary artery stenosis. J Interv Cardiol 2003;16:171–88.

7. Formigari R, Santoro G, Guccione P, et al. Treatment of pulmonary artery stenosis after arterial switch operation: stent implantation vs. balloon angioplasty. Catheter Cardiovasc Interv 2000;50(2): 207–11.

8. Geggel RL, Gauvreau K, Lock JE. Balloon dilation angioplasty of peripheral pulmonary stenosis associated with Williams syndrome. Circulation 2018;103: 2165–70.

9. Chen Q, Ma K, Hua Z, et al. Multistage pulmonary artery rehabilitation in patients with pulmonary atresia, ventricular septal defect and hypoplastic pulmonary artery. Eur J Cardiothorac Surg 2016;50(1):160–6.

Current Transcatheter Approaches for the Treatment of Aortic Coarctation in Children and Adults

Sarosh P. Batlivala, MD, MSCI, Bryan H. Goldstein, MD*

KEYWORDS

- Coarctation • Balloon aortic angioplasty • Balloon-expandable stent delivery • Covered stents

KEY POINTS

- Native coarctation of the aorta, especially in adolescents and adults, is treated with balloon-expandable stents as first-line therapy.
- Recurrent (ie, postintervention) coarctation can occasionally be treated successfully with balloon angioplasty alone.
- All patients are prone to aneurysm formation and recurrent coarctation, so lifelong follow-up with a congenital cardiologist is recommended.
- Covered stents are used to exclude aneurysms and provide additional safety; they are also used as emergency treatment of vessel disruption after balloon angioplasty/bare-metal stent placement.

INTRODUCTION

Coarctation of the aorta is an obstructive lesion characterized by congenital narrowing of the aorta. This narrowing typically occurs in the proximal descending aorta, near the insertion of the patent ductus arteriosus (PDA),[1] although the anatomy can vary. The specific anatomic characteristics can differ widely with discrete versus "long-segment" variations, associated hypoplasia of the transverse arch, and the development of severe aortic tortuosity and post-stenotic aneurysms in older patients. This clinical variability contributes to therapeutic challenges.

Aortic coarctation is a fairly common form of congenital heart disease (CHD), accounting for approximately 4% to 8% of all CHD with a prevalence of 4 per 10,000 live births.[2]

There is a male predominance, with male/female ratios ranging from approximately 1.3 to 1.7.[3] Some genetic syndromes are associated with coarctation (eg, Turner syndrome), but most cases are in nonsyndromic patients. Although first described in the 1700s, the first operations for coarctation were performed in 1944 (independently by Drs Gross and Crafood) and the first balloon angioplasty considerably later in 1978.[4,5] With incremental improvement in technique and equipment, percutaneous interventions for coarctation have become first-line therapy for most patients outside of infancy and early childhood.[6] This article summarizes the current state-of-the-art of transcatheter therapies for native and recurrent coarctation of the aorta.

Disclosure Statement: None.

The Heart Institute, Cincinnati Children's Hospital Medical Center, 3333 Burnet Avenue, Cincinnati, OH 45229, USA
* Corresponding author.
E-mail address: bryan.goldstein@cchmc.org

DIAGNOSIS

Coarctation was classically described as having a bimodal distribution (ie, infantile and adult-onset types), but more recent data have demonstrated that the disease can present at any age (Fig. 1). The most severe forms are termed "critical" because the patient requires a PDA to maintain systemic circulation. Critical variants of aortic coarctation may be diagnosed in utero with fetal echocardiography, which is more common when coarctation is identified or suspected in the setting for additional CHD lesions. Alternatively, critical coarctation in the neonate may be suspected on encountering the classic findings of a murmur (systolic or continuous, loudest in interscapular region), diminished lower extremity pulses, decreased urine output, tachypnea, and poor feeding.[1] These symptoms develop after the PDA becomes restrictive or closes, which in turn leads to decreased systemic cardiac output and inadequate peripheral perfusion. Noncritical forms of coarctation often present later, most commonly with upper-extremity hypertension with or without a systolic murmur. For this reason, all patients diagnosed with hypertension should be screened for coarctation with four-extremity blood pressure measurements. Older patients can also present with headaches, an abnormal screening electrocardiogram with left ventricular hypertrophy, or a murmur.[3] Bicuspid aortic valve is commonly associated with coarctation of the aorta and should thus be screened for with echocardiography in all patients. Fig. 2 outlines a common sequence of diagnosis and testing.

PROGNOSIS AND COMPLICATIONS

The prognosis for patients with isolated coarctation of the aorta, including the critical variants, is generally excellent given currently effective treatment strategies. With the implementation of screening programs for critical CHD in nearly all states, late diagnoses presenting in extremis and cardiogenic shock are rare. The immediate post-procedure survival for surgical and percutaneous interventions is approximately 98% to 99% for uncomplicated coarctation.[6] Nevertheless, patients with coarctation (even when successfully treated) are at risk for development of systemic hypertension, altered exercise capacity, early coronary artery disease, and ventricular dysfunction.[7]

Complications from coarctation of the aorta typically relate to incomplete treatment or to the intervention itself. Untreated critical

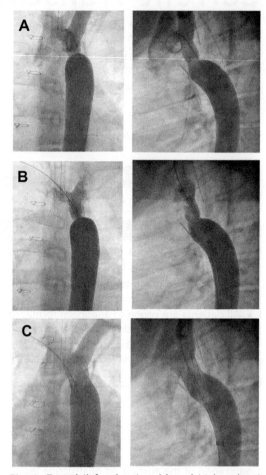

Fig. 1. Frontal (*left column*) and lateral (*right column*) angiograms of a 17-year-old patient status post-VSD and -PDA repair as an infant, subsequently diagnosed with coarctation at age 10 but lost to follow-up. (*A*) Aortic angiography demonstrates the site of long-segment coarctation at the aortic isthmus, with the adjacent surgical clip located at the site of the PDA. Note the presence of post-stenotic dilatation in the proximal descending aorta, before the aorta tapers to its "normal" caliber adjacent to the diaphragm (not seen). (*B*) Aortography documenting positioning of a bare-metal 3110 Palmaz XL stent, mounted on an 18 mm × 3.5 cm balloon-in-balloon (NuMED, Hopkinton, NY) catheter, across the site of coarctation, before stent implantation. Wire position is in the right subclavian artery. (*C*) Aortography after deployment of the stent, demonstrating a significantly improved isthmus diameter, now measuring ~2 mm smaller than the normal descending aorta at the diaphragm. The bare metal stent protrudes only minimally across the origin of the left subclavian artery. No acute aortic wall injury is present.

congenital coarctation can lead to multiple complications if not diagnosed early, including the development of cardiogenic shock, end-organ dysfunction, and death. Coarctation that is not

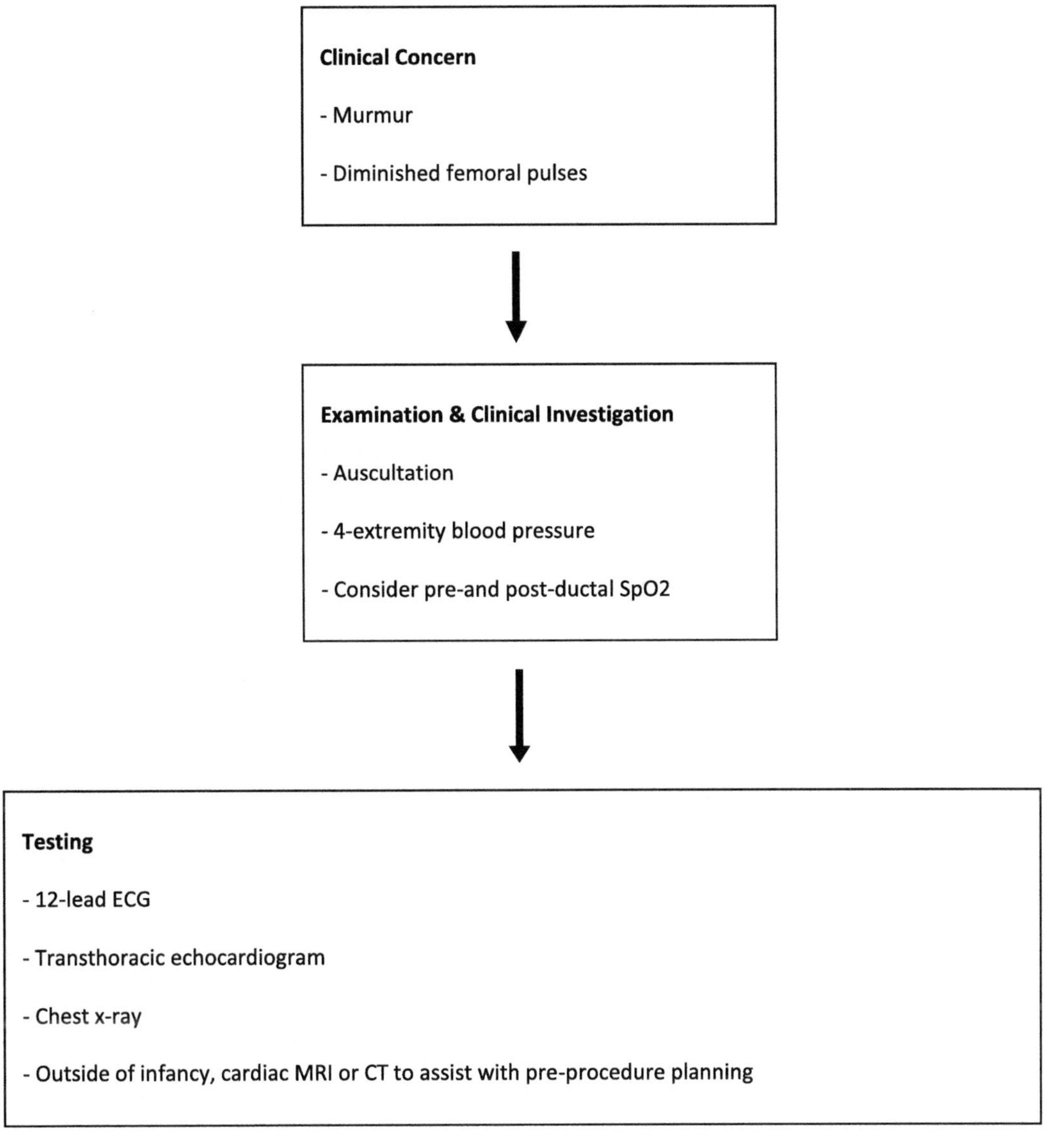

Fig. 2. Diagnostic algorithm for coarctation of the aorta. CT, computed tomography; ECG, electrocardiogram; Sp_{O2}, oxygen saturation as measured by pulse oximetry.

diagnosed until young adulthood or adulthood is associated with chronic precoarctation (upper extremity) hypertension, and as such is associated with a significantly increased risk of stroke and early coronary artery disease. Left ventricular hypertrophy with subsequent left ventricular dysfunction can also develop as a consequence of untreated aortic obstruction. Following treatment of coarctation, long-term hypertension may still result, especially if the repair was not completed until after age 8 to 9 years. Local aortic wall injury, including late aneurysm formation, is also a well-described complication. Lastly, there is an association between coarctation and berry aneurysms,[8] which increases the risk of intracranial hemorrhage in this population, and may justify routine screening with noninvasive cerebral imaging.

CLINICAL MANAGEMENT

Management of patients with coarctation depends on age at presentation and overall severity of the lesion. A detailed discussion of medical management is not described herein, given the myriad presentations of coarctation ranging from cardiogenic shock to asymptomatic hypertension. Surgical repair remained the only form of intervention from 1945 until the advent of balloon aortic angioplasty reported in 1982.[9] Percutaneous techniques have evolved rapidly with continuous advancement in sheath, balloon, and stent technology, which have progressively allowed for passage of larger diameter equipment through smaller diameter access sheaths. In the current era, percutaneous intervention is generally the procedure of choice for older school age, adolescent, and adult patients with native coarctation and those with recurrent coarctation, although surgical repair may still be performed in some centers.[10]

Although some operators attempt angioplasty first, balloon-expandable stent implantation is currently regarded as standard-of-care therapy for adolescent and adult patients with coarctation of the aorta. While balloon angioplasty may be effective in certain cases, the elastic nature of the aorta results in the need for oversizing of the angioplasty balloon beyond the diameter of nearby "normal" aorta. This nature of angioplasty, thus, makes it more likely to be associated with long-term complications, including incomplete relief of obstruction and aortic wall injury, including aneurysm. Aortic stent implantation is recognized as the most effective minimally invasive therapeutic intervention for selected patients with native coarctation of the aorta. Recurrent, or postoperative, coarctation, however, can often be treated successfully with balloon angioplasty alone, especially in the case of early recurrent obstruction. Late recurrence of aortic obstruction typically requires stent placement for relief.

TECHNIQUES
Preprocedure Testing
Preprocedure testing varies across practices. Common precatheterization testing includes a complete blood count, type-and-cross match, chest radiograph, and electrocardiogram. Echocardiography is typically obtained at the time of diagnosis, but may be inadequate to visualize the entirety of the arch, especially in adolescent or adult patients. Ascertainment of four-extremity blood pressures is a necessity, to define indications for intervention and long-term follow-up postintervention. The addition of cross-sectional imaging, including either cardiac MRI or axial computed tomography, is extraordinarily helpful in preprocedural planning for select patients. Cross-sectional imaging can help determine the precise length of the lesion; diameters of nearby "normal" aorta; assess for the presence of transverse arch hypoplasia; and provide data on the location of adjacent structures, such as the airway.[11] High-quality imaging can facilitate accurate preprocedural

planning with regards to equipment selection (balloon and stent sizes), interventional wire position, ideal fluoroscopic angles, and nearby landmarks. Stress testing may be obtained in certain occasions to evaluate for the development of systemic hypertension, and/or arm-leg blood pressure gradient accentuation during exercise.

Invasive Diagnostic Assessment
A standard right and left heart catheterization is typically performed via a femoral approach.[12–14] The case is started with procedural sedation, based on institutional practice and patient needs. Ultrasound-guided vascular access is especially helpful given the often poor femoral pulses, and pathologic consequences to an "atypical" arteriotomy site, given the large diameter arterial sheath that is used. The right heart catheterization is useful because longstanding coarctation may be associated with left ventricular dysfunction and secondary left atrial and pulmonary hypertension. We also recommend assessing for an interatrial communication, even if there is no evidence on noninvasive imaging, by simple probing of the atrial septum. Although not crucial, transatrial access to the left heart can allow for placement of an angiographic catheter in the ascending aorta, which is used to measure a precise, concomitant pressure gradient across the coarctation, throughout the procedure. A catheter in this position also allows for angiographic interrogate before, during, and immediately after the intervention. That said, access to the left heart is not mandatory, although some operators do perform a trans septal puncture for the previously stated reasons. Lastly, assessment of cardiac output is essential in the interpretation of systolic coarctation gradients, which may be diminished in the setting of low cardiac output.

Angiography is generally performed with a pigtail catheter in the aorta, immediately proximal to the aortic lesion. Biplane interrogation is highly recommended, but not absolutely mandatory, for treatment of aortic coarctation. We deliver a power-injection of 1 mL/kg (maximum 30–40 mL) over 1 second. We are careful to avoid significant contrast reflux retrograde into the ascending aorta because this can obscure the area of interest. A 20° to 30° left anterior oblique angulation on the "A" plane camera (in the setting of a left-sided aortic arch) with straight lateral angulation on the "B" plane provides an acceptable initial angiogram in most cases. The left anterior oblique angulation helps offset the ascending and descending aorta to better visualize the narrowed segment. The operator can fine-tune the angulation based on the preprocedural cross-sectional imaging and the initial screening angiogram.

Balloon Aortic Angioplasty

Aortic angioplasty as a definitive therapy is generally reserved for postoperative coarctation recurrence and select, milder forms of nonneonatal discrete coarctation.[12–14] Angioplasty may also be used in neonatal coarctation as palliative therapy, when definitive surgery is contraindicated. We have a few recommendations to perform in preparation for successful angioplasty. First, aortic angioplasty is painful and so we opt to convert to general anesthesia if the initial hemodynamics were obtained under sedation or local anesthetic. Once under general anesthesia, the sheath is upsized based on the characteristics of the intended balloon dilation catheters. Consideration should be given to use of a vascular closure device at this point, as some suture-based closure strategies require pre-placement, prior to large bore sheath insertion. Finally, ensure that an adequate selection of bare-metal and covered stents are readily available in case of vessel injury, including dissection or rupture.

Consider placement of a long sheath before any aortic interventions. The long sheath allows for rapid postdilation angiography to assess the efficacy of the dilation, and for vascular injury or disruption. A 0.035-inch guidewire is first placed in either the aortic root or subclavian artery, contralateral to the arch sidedness. Given the fairly straight catheter course, a medium stiff wire generally provides sufficient support for angioplasty and stent delivery, although stiffer wires may be required. Following angiography, a balloon is selected based on the minimal diameter of the coarctation and the sizes of the "normal" aorta immediately proximal to the coarctation and at the level of the diaphragm. Remember that many cases develop poststenotic dilation, so the area immediately distal to the coarctation should not be used as a reference for normal aortic diameter. In general, we select an initial balloon that is the lesser of 90% to 100% of the normal aortic dimension or two times the minimal diameter. We initially use a medium-pressure balloon and may progress to higher pressure non-compliant balloons based on the balloon characteristics during inflation (ie, waist/balloon ratio, compliance of the lesion). Angiography is repeated after each balloon dilation to assess the response of the vessel and to evaluate for vessel injury. Balloon/aortic ratio

may exceed 100%, even reaching 120% in some cases, to achieve an adequate result. We define success as trivial residual gradient ($\leq$10 mm Hg) without significant vessel wall damage.

Balloon-Expandable Stent Implantation for Coarctation of the Aorta

Angioplasty is often ineffective given aortic elasticity. Even when acutely effective, the durability of balloon aortic angioplasty is limited by restenosis (15%–20% of patients) and aneurysm formation (~5% of patients).[12–14] Therefore balloon-expandable stent implantation has emerged as a mainstay of transcatheter coarctation therapy. Aside from emergent and extreme situations, most interventionalists limit aortic stent placement to older children and adolescents. Doing so allows for safe passage of an adequate-sized femoral artery sheath, facilitates use of a stent capable of future dilation to normal aortic dimensions, and ensures large initial stent implant diameter, thereby extending the interval until subsequent redilation is indicated to match somatic growth in still growing patients.

A stent's radial strength opposes aortic wall recoil, may improve vessel integrity following the trauma inherent to angioplasty, and avoids the need for balloon overdilation (eg, the balloon/aortic ratio should not exceed 100%) of the adjacent normal aorta, thereby decreasing the risk of aneurysm formation at the dilation site. Most congenital interventional cardiologists use the Palmaz Genesis XD/XL line of Cordis (Milpitas, CA) stents or the Intra-Stent LD line of Medtronic stents (Minneapolis, MN).[15–17] Both of these stent families consist of large-diameter stents that can reach adult size. The Palmaz genesis stents are closed-cell design and have slightly higher radial force characteristics than the Medtronic stents (formerly EV3). That said, the open-cell design Medtronic/EV3 stents provide ample radial force for coarctation, better conform to anatomic curves, and allow for postimplant side-hole dilation (if operating in the region of a brachiocephalic vessel), prompting many operators to elect this stent family. These stent models must be hand-crimped onto an angioplasty balloon. In general, we prefer balloon-in-balloon (BIB) catheters (NuMED, Hopkinton, NY) to deploy the stent. The BIB balloons provide for a more controlled inflation, because angiograms can be obtained after inflating the inner balloon to fine-tune the stent position; they are also associated with less stent shortening. In terms of delivery, some operators opt to rapidly pace the right ventricular in patients to reduce stroke volume and thereby increase the stability and precision of the stent deployment. As with angioplasty, an immediate postdeployment angiogram is obtained to assess the intervention and evaluate for vascular injury. A covered stent should be available in the event of a dissection or vessel disruption. We assess for recoil by monitoring balloon deflation via fluoroscopy. The stent is often postdilated with a higher-pressure balloon (eg, Z-med II, B. Braun Medical Inc, Bethlehem, PA; Atlas, Bard, Tempe, AZ) if residual obstruction persists.

The availability of covered stents has provided additional safety for transcatheter therapies. Some patients with coarctation have vulnerable aortic walls, including those with Turner syndrome and older adults, among others. The covered CP stents (NuMED) were developed years ago, but have only recently been approved for use in the United States by the Food and Drug Administration. These stents are comprised of a bare-metal CP stent with an expandable polytetrafluoroethylene covering. The stents are provided in 8 zig and 10 zig designs, range in length from 16 mm to 60 mm and are dilatable up to a diameter of 24 to 30 mm, which is adequate for nearly all patients at adult-size. Complete details for these stents can be reviewed at: http://www.numedfor children.com/cpstent-fda.htm.

EVIDENCE
Balloon Angioplasty
Balloon angioplasty has been performed for native coarctation, with many studies demonstrating reasonable acute success ranging from 80% to nearly 100%.[18,19] The procedure is safe with no procedural mortality reported in a registry review of 143 patients.[20,21] However, the acute outcomes for neonates were significantly less impressive with lower acute efficacy and higher reintervention rates, probably caused by the presence of ductal tissue (rather than fibrotic scar) in this population.[20] Furthermore, data have demonstrated that long-term durability of balloon angioplasty alone is suboptimal with recent studies demonstrating a nearly 55% reintervention rate.[22] As a result, few operators perform balloon angioplasty alone for native coarctation.

As opposed to native coarctation, data are convincing that recurrent coarctation does respond effectively to balloon angioplasty. In fact, the American Heart Association supports treating recurrent coarctation with balloon angioplasty.[23] Recurrent coarctation is particularly detrimental to single ventricle patients, and a fairly large study of greater than 500 patients showed that balloon angioplasty is effective in this subset.[24] A large, multicenter prospective study comparing angioplasty for native and recurrent lesions showed that the coarct/descending aorta diameter ratio was initially higher in the recurrent coarctation intervention group compared with those who underwent native angioplasty.[21] Reobstruction after angioplasty was infrequent during early follow-up and the number of patients with trivial residual gradient (ie, <10 mm Hg) actually decreased from the early to intermediate follow-up periods in the recurrent angioplasty group, suggesting ongoing beneficial aortic remodeling. Furthermore, native angioplasty patients had a higher proportion of postdilation aneurysms and wall injury.[19] However, recurrent obstruction rates were similar between the native and recurrent coarctation angioplasty groups at intermediate follow-up.[21] Long-term data from other studies demonstrate that the incidence of recurrence requiring another intervention is as high as 50%.[22,25]

Stent Placement
Multiple animal studies have demonstrated that balloon-expandable stent placement is acutely effective in experimental models of coarctation. A small study of dogs demonstrated that stent implantation was acutely effective and safe.[26,27] Pathologic examination of the dogs' aortas demonstrated neointimal covering with an endothelial cell surface. Additional animal work has also demonstrated that coarctation stents are safely and effectively redilated.[28,29]

Numerous clinical studies have also been performed and document the effectiveness and relative safety of transcatheter stent placement for treatment of coarctation of the aorta in humans.[30–34] Stent therapy can benefit patients with native and recurrent postoperative coarctation with equal effectiveness and acceptable safety. Early clinical studies in humans used bare-metal stainless steel stents and, similar to the animal data, demonstrated that stenting was acutely effective, reducing gradients to less than 10 mm Hg in most patients, which was shown to be durable for at least 2 years.[35] The Coarctation of the Aorta Stent Trials (COAST) I was a landmark study in this regard, demonstrating that bare-metal stents were safe and effective for the treatment of coarctation.[36] As in animals, angiography demonstrated mild neointimal growth in approximately 30% of patients at 2 years. Small aneurysms occurred in approximately 7% to 10% of patients and were successfully treated with coil implantation.[21,35]

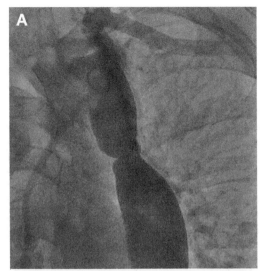

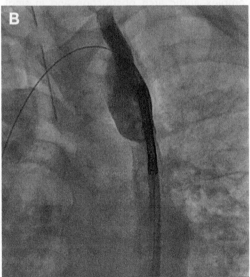

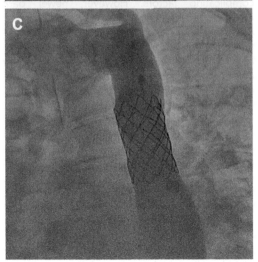

Forbes and colleagues,[33] as part of the Congenital Cardiovascular Interventional Study Consortium, reported one of the largest series of coarctation stenting to date. A total of 565 stent procedures were performed for native (52%) and recurrent postoperative (48%) coarctation. Nearly all (97.9%) cases were acutely effective based on residual gradient or increase in coarctation segment diameter to greater than 0.8 of the normal aortic diameter.[37] The investigators found an era effect with regards to complications. Specifically, procedures performed before 2002 had significantly higher overall complications, although the rates of aortic complications did not significant differ. Rather, technical complications (including balloon rupture, stent migration, and presence of a cerebrovascular accident) were fewer in the more recent era, presumably reflecting technological advancement in catheter equipment and maturity of the aortic stent procedure. Importantly, the study noted that a balloon/coarctation diameter ratio exceeding 3.5 was associated with an increased risk of aortic wall pathology (eg, aneurysm) at follow-up.[33]

Covered stents are particularly effective for stenting of complex coarctation anatomy or in patients in whom the aortic wall may be more fragile, as with advancing age and certain syndromes.[38] The COAST I and II trials similarly demonstrated that covered stents are safe and effective.[36,39,40] These studies paved the road to recent Food and Drug Administration approval of these stents, and their use has been increasing since (Fig. 3).[41] Covered stents can also be useful if there is vascular damage following angioplasty or bare-metal stent placement (Fig. 4). Although not currently approved in the United States, the all-in-one NuDel system (NuMED), a premounted covered CP stent on a BIB catheter with the balloon/stent assembly

◀—————————————————

Fig. 3. Frontal angiograms in a 41-year-old patient status postcoarctation repair in infancy, now with progressive and medication-recalcitrant hypertension. (*A*) Aortic angiogram documenting moderate-to-severe recurrent coarctation, focal in nature, distal to the left subclavian artery. The narrowest segment measures 7.5 mm versus 22 mm proximal to the obstruction and at the level of the diaphragm. (*B*) Angiograms documenting positioning of a 45-mm covered CP stent mounted on a 20 mm × 3.5 cm BIB catheter (NuMED, Hopkinton, NY) across the site of coarctation. Wire position is in the aortic root. (*C*) Final angiograms after stent deployment on the 20-mm BIB, followed by postdilation with a 22-mm Atlas balloon. The stented segment diameter is now equivalent to the proximal, normal aorta. No aortic wall injury is seen.

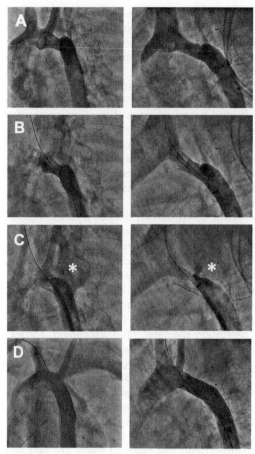

Fig. 4. Frontal (*left column*) and lateral (*right column*) angiograms of a 14-year-old patient with Turner syndrome, a bicommissural aortic valve, and aortic coarctation status postsurgical coarctation repair in infancy with the left subclavian flap technique. (*A*) Baseline angiography demonstrating significant long-segment recurrent coarctation. The left subclavian is not visualized to arise from the aorta. (*B*) Positioning of a 3110 Palmaz XL stent, mounted on a 14 mm × 3.5 cm BIB balloon. (*C*) Angiography after deployment of the Palmaz stent is notable for an acute aortic wall injury, with contrast extravasation into the tissue posterosuperiorly (*asterisk*). (*D*) Angiogram after rapid delivery and implantation of a 31-mm premounted CP covered stent. There is no significant residual coarctation and the aortic wall injury has been excluded (covered) with no evidence of persistent aortic wall injury.

preloaded into a long sheath, is particularly useful in emergency situations.[42]

In addition to native and recurrent coarctation, transcatheter stent therapy may also be a reasonable strategy for patients in whom surgery poses an unacceptably high risk or who have anatomic variants that create significant surgical difficulty (Fig. 5). Coarctation with hypoplasia of the transverse aortic arch is one

example (Fig. 6), because it can lead to clinically meaningful residual obstruction and associated long-term complications after surgical repair of simple coarctation alone.[43,44] The risks of comprehensive arch surgery (treating the coarctation and arch hypoplasia) are greater than for isolated coarctation, because the technique usually requires hypothermic circulatory arrest. A few series have reported the successful use of stent therapy for transverse arch hypoplasia. The procedure was successful in all reported cases, with anatomic and hemodynamic relief of arch obstruction.[45,46] Rigorous interrogation of stent therapy for treatment of transverse arch hypoplasia, including procedural risks and long-term outcomes, has not been undertaken.

Stent placement has also been reported for complex aortic arch obstruction and in single ventricle patients after the Norwood operation.[47,48] Novel delivery techniques, including hybrid per-aortic approach (via sternotomy) and percutaneous or cut-down facilitated carotid or axillary artery access, have been used in smaller patients to facilitate larger profile stent delivery and avoid femoral arterial injury, which is a major source of morbidity and mortality.[48,49] These children require subsequent catheterizations for stent redilation to match somatic growth.

Given considerable improvement in equipment and technique, the risk-to-benefit ratio has slowly shifted such that some cardiologists favor percutaneous therapy in milder forms of coarctation. We presume few physicians would recommend surgery for a mild coarctation with less than 20 mm Hg resting systolic gradient, in the absence of complicating factors. However, newer data demonstrate that milder forms of coarctation are associated with prolonged systemic arterial hypertension, altered exercise indices, and left ventricular hypertrophy and diastolic dysfunction.[7] Early data regarding stent therapy for treatment of mild coarctation demonstrated acute success with no significant residual gradient at follow-up, slight improvement in left ventricular end-diastolic pressure (median, 17–14 mm Hg), and improvement in exercise capacity, suggesting potential benefit to diastolic function and overall cardiovascular fitness.[30,50] However, other studies have found that late aneurysm formation, systemic hypertension, left ventricular stroke work, and aortic wall shear stress forces were not associated with mild chronic residual aortic obstruction.[51,52] As is often the case with evolving therapies, larger clinical studies with longer term follow-up will help determine if treatment of mild disease is beneficial

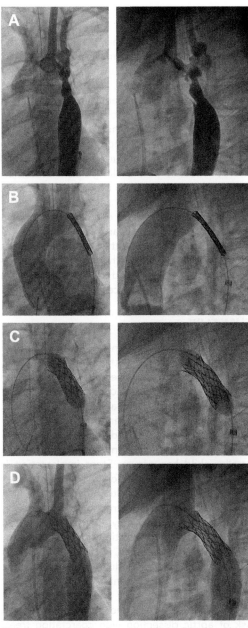

and justifies the risks of the procedure and its long-term sequelae. For now, we urge caution in treatment of this population.

CONTROVERSIES

The treatment of smaller patients (<20–25 kg) with significant coarctation using stent therapy remains a source of substantial controversy within the field, because the implanted stent should ideally be dilatable (at subsequent procedures) to adult size. Stents capable of large-diameter dilation require larger profile delivery sheaths, which compromise the femoral-iliac arterial system at this size. A "growth stent" was developed to help deal with this issue. The growth stent is comprised of two longitudinal stent-halves that are connected by bioresorbable sutures to create a complete cylindrical stent that is implanted.[53] These stents were acutely successful and were able to be dilated as expected. However, pathologic specimens from animal studies demonstrated thinning of the aortic wall in the portions of the aorta between the stent halves.[54] This stent was not approved in the United States and never gained substantial traction. The literature does suggest that standard stents can subsequently be delivered to further treat residual obstruction related to somatic growth, but this requires implantation of a large-diameter-capable stent.[55]

Beyond the issue of technical feasibility, placement of an aortic stent in a school-age child incurs the need for at least one subsequent catheterization to further dilate the stent to match growth. Surgical repair in this age group, although potentially more morbid than transcatheter stent implantation, results in definitive coarctation therapy with one procedure, in most cases. Of course, many cardiologists still recommend percutaneous intervention, arguing that two percutaneous procedures (generally with only an overnight hospital stay each time) is less burdensome than even a single operation and hospital stay. This position may be further enhanced by long-term operative data suggesting

Fig. 5. Frontal (*left column*) and lateral (*right column*) angiograms of 13-year-old patient presenting with headaches, diagnosed with native coarctation. (*A*) Initial angiography documents severe and bizarre coarctation beginning just distal to the left common carotid artery. Both the distal aorta and the proximal left subclavian artery have multiple aneurysms present, with slow transit of contrast to the left upper extremity. There is also a tiny PDA present, with prominent post-stenotic dilation of the adjacent descending aorta. (*B*) Following considerable and multidisciplinary discussions about the ideal therapeutic strategy, a 39-mm covered stent is advanced into position to cover the origins of the diseased left subclavian artery (LSCA) and PDA. Distal wire rests looped in the aortic root. (*C*) Image of the stent inflation on a 14-mm BIB catheter (NuMED, Hopkinton, NY); note the waists at the level of the LSCA and the aortic isthmus. (*D*) Final angiography after stent implantation; the segment is notably wider and the PDA and LSCA are covered (although not seen in this still angiogram, the LSCA fills retrograde via the ipsilateral vertebral artery); the distal stent extends minimally into the area of post-stenotic dilation, ensuring the entire segment is treated.

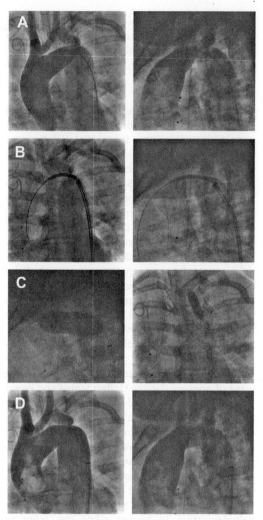

The advent of bioresorbable stents may only further this controversy. Bioresorbable stents are currently investigational in this domain, but may soon be available in small sizes (and delivery profiles) capable of being used to treat neonatal and infantile coarctation. Various stents have been developed with differing resorption times, ranging from 2 months to more than a year.[57] No data yet exist about their use in this population (beyond a few isolated case reports), which needs to include procedural complications and short-, medium-, and long-term outcomes. Patient selection needs to be defined. This population and therapy could set-up well for a prospective device trial in coarctation requiring therapy less than 1 year of age. Some researchers hypothesize that bioresorbable stents may be used in infancy with subsequent percutaneous bare-metal/covered stent intervention in late childhood/adolescence as indicated.

SUMMARY

Transcatheter coarctation intervention, most frequently performed with stent implantation, is an effective and still evolving approach to the treatment of native and postoperative recurrent coarctation of the aorta. Most pediatric interventionalists limit coarctation stent implantation to large children and adolescents to avoid the need for aortic stent redilation when a smaller child has grown. Stent implantation is frequently a viable solution for more complex coarctation anatomy, including transverse arch hypoplasia and arch obstruction after the Norwood operation, and may even be considered in milder forms of coarctation that have not warranted surgery in the past, although this remains controversial. In older adults where the aortic wall is friable, covered stents may provide a safer alternative to traditional angioplasty of bare-metal stent placement, because of the increased risk of aortic dissection with coarctation treatment. Longer-term follow-up studies are necessary to more precisely define the late risks of stent restenosis, aortic aneurysm formation, stent redilation to match somatic growth in children, and blood pressure response to exercise in the face of a rigid, stented aortic segment.

Fig. 6. Frontal (*left column*) and lateral (*right column*) angiograms of a 41-year-old patient diagnosed with arch obstruction as a teenager, although no prior interventions were performed. (*A*) Baseline angiography demonstrates transverse aortic arch hypoplasia, with the narrowest segment just after the take-off of the left subclavian artery (LSCA) and post-stenotic dilation of the proximal descending aorta. (*B*) Positioning of a 36-mm EV3 LD Max (Medtronic, Minneapolis, MN) stent hand-crimped onto a 22 mm × 4 cm BIB catheter (NuMED, Hopkinton, NY). Note that the origin of the LSCA is intentionally crossed to ensure adequate stent treatment of the transverse arch. (*C*) Image of the stent inflation with stable stent position across the transverse arch (*left*). Subsequent dilation of the LSCA origin using a 10-mm balloon to prevent metal stent struts from crossing the LSCA origin (*right*). (*D*) Angiography after deployment of the stent demonstrates marked improvement in the transverse arch diameter with unobstructed flow into the LSCA.

that approximately 10% of patients who undergo initial operative repair of coarctation require a subsequent percutaneous intervention for recurrence of aortic obstruction.[56]

REFERENCES

1. Keane JF, Lock JE, Fyler DC, et al. Nadas' pediatric cardiology. 2nd edition. Philadelphia: Saunders; 2006.
2. Hoffman JIE, Kaplan S. The incidence of congenital heart disease. J Am Coll Cardiol 2002;39(12): 1890–900.

3. Moss AJ, Allen HD. Ch. 36 - aortic arch anomalies. In: Moss and Adams' heart disease in infants, children, and adolescents: including the fetus and young adult. Philadelphia: Wolters Kluwer Health/ Lippincott Williams & Wilkins; 2008.

4. Crafoor C, Nylin G. Congenital coarctation of the aorta and its surgical treatment. J Thorac Cardiovasc Surg 1945;14:347–61.

5. Gross R, Hufnagel C. Coarctation of the aorta. Experimental studies regarding its surgical correction. N Engl J Med 1945;233(10):287–93.

6. Zussman ME, Hirsch R, Herbert C, et al. Transcatheter intervention for coarctation of the aorta. Cardiol Young 2016;26(8):1563–7.

7. Dijkema EJ, Leiner T, Grotenhuis HB. Diagnosis, imaging and clinical management of aortic coarctation. Heart 2017;103(15):1148–55.

8. Taylor CL, Yuan Z, Selman WR, et al. Cerebral arterial aneurysm formation and rupture in 20,767 elderly patients: hypertension and other risk factors. J Neurosurg 1995;83(5):812–9.

9. Singer MI, Rowen M, Dorsey TJ. Transluminal aortic balloon angioplasty for coarctation of the aorta in the newborn. Am Heart J 1982;103(1):131–2.

10. Hijazi ZM, Awad SM. Pediatric cardiac interventions. JACC Cardiovasc Interv 2008;1(6):603–11.

11. Gach P, Dabadie A, Sorensen C, et al. Multimodality imaging of aortic coarctation: From the fetus to the adolescent. Diagn Interv Imaging 2016;97(5): 581–90.

12. Bergersen L, Foerster S, Marshall A, et al. Congenital heart disease: the catheterization manual. New York: Springer; 2009.

13. Mullins CE. Cardiac catheterization in congenital heart disease: pediatric and adult. 1st edition. Malden (MA): Blackwell Publishing; 2006.

14. Sievert H, Qureshi SA, Wilson N, et al. Percutaneous interventions for congenital heart disease. London: Informa Healthcare; 2007.

15. Ebeid M. Balloon expandable stents for coarctation of the aorta: review of current status and technical considerations. Images Paediatr Cardiol 2003;5(2): 25–41.

16. Medtronic/EV3 stent info. Available at: https:// www.medtronic.com/us-en/healthcare-professionals/ products/cardiovascular/peripheral-biliary-stents/ intrastent-max-ld-biliary-stent.html. Accessed May 15, 2018.

17. Palmaz stent information. Available at: https://emea. cordis.com/emea/endovascular/lower-extremity-solutions/intervene/balloon-expandable-stents/ palmaz-genesis-peripheral-stent.html. Accessed May 15, 2018.

18. Mendelsohn AM, Lloyd TR, Crowley DC, et al. Late follow-up of balloon angioplasty in children with a native coarctation of the aorta. Am J Cardiol 1994;74(7):696–700.

19. Fawzy ME, Fathala A, Osman A, et al. Twenty-two years of follow-up results of balloon angioplasty for discreet native coarctation of the aorta in adolescents and adults. Am Heart J 2008;156(5):910–7.

20. Rao PS, Galal O, Smith PA, et al. Five- to nine-year follow-up results of balloon angioplasty of native aortic coarctation in infants and children. J Am Coll Cardiol 1996;27(2):462–70.

21. Harris KC, Du W, Cowley CG, et al, Congenital Cardiac Intervention Study Consortium (CCISC). A prospective observational multicenter study of balloon angioplasty for the treatment of native and recurrent coarctation of the aorta. Catheter Cardiovasc Interv 2014;83(7):1116–23.

22. Dijkema EJ, Sieswerda G-JT, Takken T, et al. Long-term results of balloon angioplasty for native coarctation of the aorta in childhood in comparison with surgery. Eur J Cardiothorac Surg 2018;53(1):262–8.

23. Feltes TF, Bacha E, Beekman RH, et al. Indications for cardiac catheterization and intervention in pediatric cardiac disease: a scientific statement from the American Heart Association. Circulation 2011; 123(22):2607–52.

24. Ohye RG, Sleeper LA, Mahony L, et al. Comparison of shunt types in the Norwood procedure for single-ventricle lesions. N Engl J Med 2010;362(21):1980–92.

25. Saxena A. Recurrent coarctation: interventional techniques and results. World J Pediatr Congenit Heart Surg 2015;6(2):257–65.

26. Beekman RH, Muller DW, Reynolds PI, et al. Balloon-expandable stent treatment of experimental coarctation of the aorta: early hemodynamic and pathological evaluation. J Interv Cardiol 1993;6(2):113–23.

27. Morrow WR, Smith VC, Ehler WJ, et al. Balloon angioplasty with stent implantation in experimental coarctation of the aorta. Circulation 1994;89(6):2677–83.

28. Mendelsohn AM, Dorostkar PC, Moorehead CP, et al. Stent redilation in canine models of congenital heart disease: pulmonary artery stenosis and coarctation of the aorta. Cathet Cardiovasc Diagn 1996;38(4):430–40.

29. Morrow WR, Palmaz JC, Tio FO, et al. Re-expansion of balloon-expandable stents after growth. J Am Coll Cardiol 1993;22(7):2007–13.

30. Marshall AC, Perry SB, Keane JF, et al. Early results and medium-term follow-up of stent implantation for mild residual or recurrent aortic coarctation. Am Heart J 2000;139(6):1054–60.

31. Johnston TA, Grifka RG, Jones TK. Endovascular stents for treatment of coarctation of the aorta: acute results and follow-up experience. Catheter Cardiovasc Interv 2004;62(4):499–505.

32. Shah L, Hijazi Z, Sandhu S, et al. Use of endovascular stents for the treatment of coarctation of the aorta in children and adults: immediate and midterm results. J Invasive Cardiol 2005;17(11):614–8.

33. Forbes TJ, Moore P, Pedra CAC, et al. Intermediate follow-up following intravascular stenting for treatment of coarctation of the aorta. Catheter Cardiovasc Interv 2007;70(4):569–77.

34. Mohan UR, Danon S, Levi D, et al. Stent implantation for coarctation of the aorta in children <30 kg. JACC Cardiovasc Interv 2009;2(9):877–83.

35. Suárez de Lezo J, Pan M, Romero M, et al. Immediate and follow-up findings after stent treatment for severe coarctation of aorta. Am J Cardiol 1999; 83(3):400–6.

36. Meadows J, Minahan M, McElhinney DB, et al, COAST Investigators*. Intermediate outcomes in the prospective, multicenter Coarctation of the Aorta Stent Trial (COAST). Circulation 2015; 131(19):1656–64.

37. Forbes TJ, Garekar S, Amin Z, et al. Procedural results and acute complications in stenting native and recurrent coarctation of the aorta in patients over 4 years of age: a multi-institutional study. Catheter Cardiovasc Interv 2007;70(2):276–85.

38. Varma C, Benson LN, Butany J, et al. Aortic dissection after stent dilatation for coarctation of the aorta: a case report and literature review. Catheter Cardiovasc Interv 2003;59(4):528–35.

39. Ringel RE, Vincent J, Jenkins KJ, et al. Acute outcome of stent therapy for coarctation of the aorta: results of the coarctation of the aorta stent trial. Catheter Cardiovasc Interv 2013;82(4):503–10.

40. Taggart NW, Minahan M, Cabalka AK, et al. Immediate outcomes of covered stent placement for treatment or prevention of aortic wall injury associated with Coarctation of the Aorta (COAST II). JACC Cardiovasc Interv 2016;9(5):484–93.

41. Sadiq M, Ur Rehman A, Qureshi AU, et al. Covered stents in the management of native coarctation of the aorta: intermediate and long-term follow-up. Catheter Cardiovasc Interv 2013;82(4):511–8.

42. Eicken A, Georgiev S, Ewert P. Aortic rupture during stenting for recurrent aortic coarctation in an adult: live-saving, emergency, NuDEL all-in-one covered stent implantation. Cardiol Young 2017; 27(6):1225–8.

43. Quennelle S, Powell AJ, Geva T, et al. Persistent aortic arch hypoplasia after coarctation treatment is associated with late systemic hypertension. J Am Heart Assoc 2015;4(7). https://doi.org/10.1161/JAHA.115.001978.

44. Lu WH, Fan C-PS, Chaturvedi R, et al. Clinical impact of stent implantation for coarctation of the aorta with associated hypoplasia of the transverse aortic arch. Pediatr Cardiol 2017;38(5):1016–23.

45. Pushparajah K, Sadiq M, Brzezińska-Rajszys G, et al. Endovascular stenting in transverse aortic arch hypoplasia. Catheter Cardiovasc Interv 2013;82(4): E491–9.

46. Pihkala J, Pedra CA, Nykanen D, et al. Implantation of endovascular stents for hypoplasia of the transverse aortic arch. Cardiol Young 2000;10(1):3–7.

47. Holzer RJ, Chisolm JL, Hill SL, et al. Stenting complex aortic arch obstructions. Catheter Cardiovasc Interv 2008;71(3):375–82.

48. Aldoss O, Goldstein BH, Danon S, et al. Acute and mid-term outcomes of stent implantation for recurrent coarctation of the aorta between the Norwood operation and fontan completion: a multi-center pediatric interventional cardiology early career society investigation. Catheter Cardiovasc Interv 2017;90(6):972–9.

49. Kutty S, Burke RP, Hannan RL, et al. Hybrid aortic reconstruction for treatment of recurrent aortic obstruction after stage 1 single ventricle palliation: medium term outcomes and results of redilation. Catheter Cardiovasc Interv 2011;78(1):93–100.

50. Grøndahl C, Pedersen TAL, Hjortdal VE. The medium-term effects of treatment for mild aortic recoarctation. World J Pediatr Congenit Heart Surg 2017;8(1):55–61.

51. Keshavarz-Motamed Z, Garcia J, Kadem L. Mathematical, numerical and experimental study in the human aorta with coexisting models of bicuspid aortic stenosis and coarctation of the aorta. Conf Proc IEEE Eng Med Biol Soc 2011;2011:182–5.

52. Pedersen TAL, Munk K, Andersen NH, et al. High long-term morbidity in repaired aortic coarctation: weak association with residual arch obstruction. Congenit Heart Dis 2011;6(6):573–82.

53. Ewert P, Riesenkampff E, Neuss M, et al. Novel growth stent for the permanent treatment of vessel stenosis in growing children: an experimental study. Catheter Cardiovasc Interv 2004;62(4):506–10.

54. Sigler M, Schneider K, Meissler M, et al. Breakable stent for interventions in infants and neonates: an animal study and histopathological findings. Heart 2006;92(2):245–8.

55. Ewert P, Peters B, Nagdyman N, et al. Early and mid-term results with the Growth Stent–a possible concept for transcatheter treatment of aortic coarctation from infancy to adulthood by stent implantation? Catheter Cardiovasc Interv 2008;71(1):120–6.

56. Yetman AT, Nykanen D, McCrindle BW, et al. Balloon angioplasty of recurrent coarctation: a 12-year review. J Am Coll Cardiol 1997;30(3):811–6.

57. Nogic J, McCormick LM, Francis R, et al. Novel bioabsorbable polymer and polymer-free metallic drug-eluting stents. J Cardiol 2018; 71(5):435–43.

Transcatheter Pulmonary Valve Replacement in Congenital Heart Disease

Sanjay Sinha, MD[a],*, Jamil Aboulhosn, MD[a,b], Daniel S. Levi, MD[c]

KEYWORDS

- Transcatheter pulmonary valve replacement • Dysfunctional RVOT
- Adult congenital heart disease • Congenital heart disease

KEY POINTS

- The approved indications for transcatheter valve replacement is for replacement of dysfunctional prosthetic pulmonary valves and conduits.
- Hybrid procedures expand the use of transcatheter valves, may obviate cardiopulmonary bypass and may reduce surgical morbidity in select patients.
- Newer generation valves will expand the use of transcatheter valve replacement to the native right ventricular outflow tract.
- Long-term outcome studies are needed to assess longevity relative to surgical valves.

INTRODUCTION

Patients with dysfunctional right ventricular outflow tracks (RVOTs) comprise a large portion of patients with severe congenital heart disease.[1,2] These patients have often undergone multiple operations, and as they age, have a higher level of complexity and increase in comorbidities. They stand to benefit from minimally invasive procedures, such as transcatheter valve replacement. The technology of transcatheter valves and delivery platforms has evolved tremendously, as have the preprocedural assessment techniques, periprocedural imaging modalities, and implantation techniques needed to safely replace dysfunctional valves. This review discusses the approach and preprocedural planning, current options, and applications of transcatheter pulmonary valve therapy; touches on future directions; and expounds on the techniques used for implantation.

PREPROCEDURAL AND INTRAPROCEDURAL IMAGING

In the current era of transcatheter valve replacement, successful implantation in patients with acquired and congenital valvular heart disease is predicated on a thorough assessment of the "landing zone," the behavior of the valve in the target environment, and interaction with the surrounding structures/tissues. The radial force, and compliance of an RVOT after a transannular patch repair, for example, differ in its interaction with a transcatheter valve delivery as compared with a calcified homograft conduit. Given the potential for complications, such as valve embolization, paravalvular regurgitation, and vascular injury, it is essential to gain information and understanding of these variables before valve implantation to maximize the safety and efficacy of the procedure. This is achieved with multimodality preprocedural planning that includes:

Disclosure Statement: Dr J. Aboulhosn is a proctor for Medtronic and Edwards Lifesciences.
[a] Department of Pediatrics, Division of Cardiology, UCLA Mattel Children's Hospital, Los Angeles, CA, USA; [b] Department of Medicine, Division of Cardiology, Ahmanson/UCLA Adult Congenital Heart Disease Center, Ronald Reagan UCLA Medical Center, 100 Medical Plaza, Suite 630E, Los Angeles, CA 90024, USA; [c] Division of Cardiology, UCLA Mattel Children's Hospital, University of California Los Angeles Medical School, 200 UCLA Medical Plaza #330, Los Angeles, CA 90095, USA
* Corresponding author. 200 Medical Plaza, Suite 224, Los Angeles, CA 90024.
E-mail address: ssinha@mednet.ucla.edu

Intervent Cardiol Clin 8 (2019) 59–71
https://doi.org/10.1016/j.iccl.2018.08.006
2211-7458/19/© 2018 Elsevier Inc. All rights reserved.

1. Cross-sectional imaging with computed tomography angiography (CTA) (preferably electrocardiogram [ECG] gated) or cardiac MRI
2. Multiplanar reconstruction and three-dimensional (3D) reconstruction of cross-sectional imaging
3. Consideration of ex vivo bench testing of 3D-printed models
4. Echocardiography with Doppler

CROSS-SECTIONAL IMAGING

Before the index procedure, cross-sectional imaging is used to comprehensively assess the valve landing zone.[3,4] The ideal study should provide high temporal and spatial resolution throughout the cardiac cycle; ECG-gated CTA is ideal for this indication with spatial resolution between 0.3 and 0.7 mm. Protocols that include abdominal and pelvic arterial imaging are imperative for assessment of patients considering transcatheter aortic valve replacement.[3] These studies are done rapidly and do not require sedation for patients, and may be performed in those with implantable pacemakers and other metallic devices. The main limitation of this modality is the inevitable exposure to ionizing radiation; this is an especially important consideration in patients with congenital heart disease (CHD), many of whom have been or will be exposed to numerous radiation-based diagnostic and interventional procedures throughout their life.[5,6]

MRI technology has advanced significantly and offers some significant benefits in preprocedural planning. MRI can provide volumetric data required to assess the indications for valve replacement in regards to ventricular ejection fraction, regurgitant fraction, systolic and diastolic volumetric data, and flow quantification.[7,8] High-fidelity MRI with newer contrast agents, such as intravenous iron, allows for a study that highlights the entire blood pool (venous and arterial systems), does not expose the patient to radiation, and does not subject the patient to traditional iodine- or gadolinium-based contrast agents. These studies can also provide dynamic assessment of valvular, ventricular, and vascular motion and changes thereof throughout the cardiac cycle. Assessment of the venous and arterial access patency is safely visualized without the need for extraionizing radiation before the index procedure. Patients with pacemakers and other metallic implants may suffer from magnetic artifacts that can adversely affect anatomic assessment and this is unfortunately an ongoing limitation of MRI.

MULTIPLANAR RECONSTRUCTION AND THREE-DIMENSIONAL RECONSTRUCTION

Either modality provides cross-sectional volumetric data, which allows for multiplanar reconstruction using commercially available software, typically consisting of three planes (X,Y,Z) that are manually manipulated by the operator (Fig. 1A–C). Curved multiplanar reconstruction may be used to "uncoil" curving vascular structures to better assess minimum and maximum dimensions. 3D reconstruction is performed with numerous choices available for volumetric and surface rendering algorithms. The original cross-sectional data are cropped, sculpted, smoothed, and colorized as desired and areas of interest are isolated as needed (Fig. 1D).

THREE-DIMENSIONAL PRINTING AND BENCH TESTING

3D printing has become accessible and miniaturized, with many institutions and private individuals having access to high-quality printers. The steps for 3D printing involve segmenting and converting the cross-sectional imaging data to a stereolithographic file; a variety of commercially available software programs can accomplish this, the mostly widely used is Mimics (Materialise, Leuven, Belgium), which results in a "cast' of the 3D model. The 3D technician and the clinician are then able to view the model and provide further refinement to best model the patient's anatomy. The model is printed with a rapid prototyping printer and in most settings is printed on anatomically comparable material, gel-like, compliant, and translucent. Calcified regions are printed with harder and less compliant materials to mimic the tissue properties of the in vivo anatomy. With the advent of this technology, practitioners have been able to select specific thickness and compliance in the model to best approximate human arterial tissues properties (Young modulus between 0.2 and 9 MPa; pliability between 1.2×10^{-3} and 6.6×10^{-3} mm Hg) with high fidelity.[9–12] This is particularly helpful in assessing, for example, the likelihood and location of perivalvular leak in an abnormally shaped landing zone for a valve, and this type of model, therefore, can present a platform for ex vivo bench testing of an implant procedure (Fig. 2). This is now widely used in

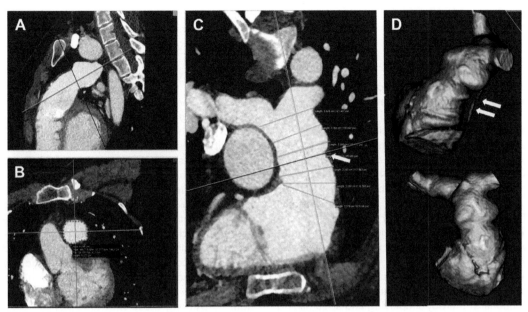

Fig. 1. Multiplanar reconstruction of an ECG-gated CTA showing a modified sagittal (*A*), axial (*B*), and RVOT view (*C*) of a patient's RVOT and pulmonary artery. This patient has a diagnosis of tetralogy of Fallot repaired using a transannular patch that has now dilated to 28.6 mm at its narrowest area (*single arrow*). The multiplanar reconstruction shows a more precise view of the potential landing zone for a transcatheter valve by opening up the anatomy in a curvilinear fashion. This can then be instantly segmented to a 3D reconstruction (*D*) and rotated, viewing only the desired structures. In this case, the RVOT and branched pulmonary arteries are shown, and the left main coronary artery to left anterior descending artery as it courses posteriorly to the pulmonary artery (*double arrow*).

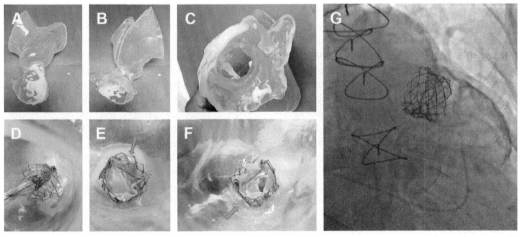

Fig. 2. 3D model and ex vivo implant of a transcatheter valve and prestent in a 68-year-man with tetralogy of Fallot status post late intracardiac repair (age 48 years old). His CTA demonstrated evidence of a calcified RVOT patch, and there was echocardiographic evidence of moderate RV enlargement, mildly reduced systolic function, moderate pulmonic regurgitation, with moderately elevated resting systolic velocity. Bench testing with a 3D printed SLA model shows the heavily calcified RVOT with a hardened opacified material printed to represent the calcium, and a soft, pliable material emulating the thickened tissue of the RVOT and pulmonary arteries (*A–C*). The Sapien XT valve was bench tested here within a Palmaz 4010 stent; however, this was shown to result in potential paravalvular leak (*arrows*) (*D–F*). This allowed for the planned placement of a Sapien S3 valve in the patient with good result and no paravalvular leak (*G*). (*Courtesy of* [Sapien XT valve] Edwards Lifesciences, Inc, Irvine, CA, with permission; and [Palmaz 4010 stent] Cordis, Inc, Fremont, CA, with permission.)

preprocedural planning for surgical and interventional CHD cases.

ECHO WITH DOPPLER

Expertise in the interpretation of preprocedural echocardiographic is imperative for appropriate selection of patients. Practitioners should also attempt to become proficient in intracardiac echocardiography (ICE), which is widely used to guide interventional procedures. ICE is a versatile modality that is ideal for imaging right-sided valves and is invaluable in the guidance of tricuspid and pulmonary valve interventions. The ICE catheter is typically advanced from the femoral vein to the right atrium or into the right ventricle (RV) and can help the interventionalist visualize the morphology of all four valves, assess for thrombi, and assess for and locate paravalvular leaks. It is controlled by the interventionalist thereby simplifying and streamlining the procedure and obviating an additional imaging specialist.[13,14] Most ICE systems require an 8F or 9F catheter sheath, which is easily tolerated in the venous system of patients greater than 30 kg, which comprise most patients undergoing transcatheter pulmonary valve replacement (TCPVR), and offers invaluable assessment of the landing zone of the valve before, and of the transcatheter valve's performance after implantation.

VALVE REPLACEMENT OPTIONS

The development of the transcatheter valve technology has revolutionized structural and congenital heart disease. The first commercially available transcatheter valve for patients with congenital heart disease was the Melody valve (Medtronic Inc, Minneapolis, MN), which was first implanted by Bonhoeffer and coworkers[15] in 2000 and received CE approval for commercial use in 2006. The Melody valve is a balloon expandable bovine jugular venous valve that was initially used for treatment of dysfunctional RV to pulmonary artery (PA) conduits, and later used for treatment of dysfunctional bioprosthetic valves and native RVOT.[16,17] A transcatheter balloon-expandable bovine pericardial valve platform for the treatment of calcific aortic stenosis was simultaneously developed and implanted in an elderly frail man with calcific aortic stenosis by Cribier in 2002.[18,19] This was the predecessor to the Sapien valve (Edwards Lifesciences, Irvine, CA), which is now in the third generation of development and is the most implanted transcatheter valve worldwide. These developments have catalyzed the rapid emergence of a host of new valves over the past 15 years, with balloon expandable and self-expanding platforms (Fig. 3).

PULMONIC VALVE REPLACEMENT

The single most common application of transcatheter valve replacement in CHD is in prosthetic pulmonary valve dysfunction, RV to PA conduit failure or the dysfunctional RVOT.[20–22] Most patients with CHD requiring TCPVR are those with repaired tetralogy of Fallot. Other etiologies include congenital pulmonary valve stenosis that has been surgically intervened on with resultant pulmonary regurgitation, those with repaired truncus arteriosus with subsequently dysfunctional RV to PA conduits, and those with congenital aortic valve pathology that have undergone the Ross operation and subsequently developed conduit dysfunction.[20,21] Among those with tetralogy of Fallot, surgical intervention in infancy is typically performed to patch the ventricular septal defect and to relieve RVOT obstruction. In those with pulmonary atresia, placement of a RV to PA conduit is typical, whereas among those with pulmonary valve stenosis surgical relief of the obstruction is achieved by dividing the annulus of the pulmonary valve and patch augmentation of the RVOT. In past decades transannular patch augmentation was widely used and therefore this surgical variant is commonly encountered in this population, resulting in predominant pulmonary regurgitation and large and often aneurysmal RVOTs. In contrast, patients that have undergone surgical conduit placement (typically using a valved aortic or pulmonic homograft) present with predominant conduit stenosis or mixed stenosis and regurgitation.[21,22] Patients with pulmonary atresia that have undergone conduit placement in infancy typically require conduit replacement during childhood and then again in late adolescence or young adulthood. Therefore, patients born with pulmonary atresia have typically undergone several surgical procedures for placement or replacement of their conduits and many older patients have eventually undergone bioprosthetic pulmonary valve replacement. The number of surgical procedures performed correlates with an increase in arrhythmia risk and risk of heart failure in adulthood, with approximately 35% of patients who have had five or more surgeries suffering from sustained ventricular tachyarrhythmias.[23] Therefore, TCPVR in these patients should be used to obviate these risks of further surgical valve replacement in the future.

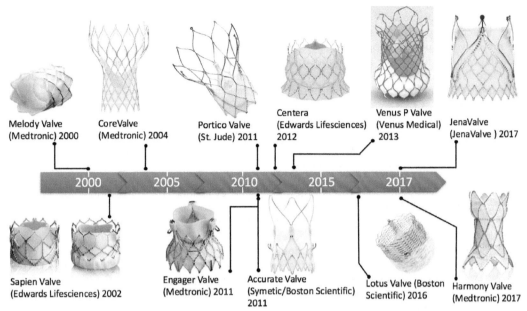

Fig. 3. Timeline of the most commonly used transcatheter valves to date. Each date represents the year the valve experienced a first-in-human implant from the first implant of the Melody valve to the JenaValve and the Harmony valve. Compared with the first decade of the millennium, the second decade has seen more than double the number of first-in-human implants. Sapien and Centera valve, included among these are also CoreValve, and Engager valve, Portico valve, the Accurate and Lotus valve, and Venus P valve. (*Courtesy of* [Melody valve] Medtronic, Inc, Minneapolis, MN, with permission; and [JenaValve] JenaValve, Inc, Irvine, CA, with permission; and [Sapien and Centera valve] Edwards Lifesciences, Inc, Irvine, CA, with permission; and [CoreValve, and Engager valve] Medtronic, with permission; and [Portico valve] Abbott, St Paul, MN, with permission; and [Accurate and Lotus valve] Image provided courtesy of Boston Scientific. © 2018 Boston Scientific Corporation or its affiliates. All rights reserved; and [Venus P valve] Venus Medtech, Hongzhou, China, with permission.)

Although the indications and timing of pulmonary valve replacement, be it surgical or transcatheter, remain controversial, it is widely accepted that those with severe stenosis and exercise limitation benefit with subsequent improvement in exercise capacity.[24] In patients with predominant pulmonary regurgitation, an indexed RV end-diastolic volume of greater than 150 mL/m² or indexed RV end-systolic volume greater than 80 mL/m² may indicate an RV that may not normalize in size after intervention; however, there are a paucity of data to suggest clinical benefit beyond improvement in RV size.[25,26] There is growing evidence suggesting that earlier pulmonary valve replacement in those with predominant PR may improve exercise tolerance and long-term benefits of RV remodeling.[24–26]

SURGICAL ANATOMY OF THE RIGHT VENTRICULAR OUTFLOW TRACT

The types of RV to PA conduits placed differ from surgeon to surgeon and era to era. Homograft material, either aortic or pulmonary, has been used extensively since 1966 and therefore

is widely encountered in these patients. Progressive dysfunction occurs in most homografts and most require replacement within 15 years of implantation if implanted in an adolescent or adult, sooner if implanted in a young child.[27,28] The mode of failure of aortic homografts is typically progressive calcification with resultant stenosis or combined stenosis and regurgitation. It is imperative for the operator to gather a comprehensive surgical history from the patient to determine the type and size of RV to PA conduit in a patient being considered for TCPVR. This is especially challenging in older patients with ACHD that may have undergone surgery decades ago without available surgical records. Heavily calcified aortic homografts are prone to dissection and rupture if dilated with high-pressure balloons beyond their original implantation size and care should be taken to dilate these conduits gradually and use covered stent platforms if possible to decrease the risk of uncontained rupture.[29] Pulmonary homografts typically are not as extensively calcified but do have a tendency to dilate with resultant regurgitation. Pulmonary homografts can often be dilated to a slightly larger diameter than the original implant diameter if deemed imperative.[30] Infective endocarditis is a serious concern and may have occurred in approximately 5% of patients with dysfunctional homografts being considered for intervention, and prior history of endocarditis is an important risk factor for endocarditis following TCPVR.[31–33] Dacron conduits are not as widely encountered in patients with ACHD and are mostly used in young children who cannot accommodate a large homograft. This material lacks distensibility and cannot be postdilated past the original implant diameter.[34] Other conduit types include the Contegra conduit (Medtronic), which is made from the bovine jugular material and comes in off-the-shelf sizes of 12 to 22 mm. This conduit uses similar material to the Melody valve but does not include stent material. Several studies have shown early failure of Contegra conduits especially with an increased RV/left ventricle pressure ratio with resultant progressive conduit dilation.[35]

BIOPROSTHETIC VALVES

Surgical placement of stented bioprosthetic valves is widely used in patients with dysfunctional conduits and native RVOTs.[36] Much like conduits, these bioprosthetic valves are destined to become dysfunctional and require replacement within 10 to 20 years of implantation. A dysfunctional bioprosthetic valve provides an ideal landing zone for TCPVR, often referred to as a valve-in-valve procedure, obviating surgical reintervention and has been done with excellent outcomes.[36,37] In the presence of undersized bioprosthetic valves that were placed in childhood, valve-in-valve can still be performed by increasing the size of the bioprosthetic valve with the use of high-pressure balloons to fracture the valve ring, typically by inflating a slightly oversized balloon (~2 mm above the published valve inner diameter and usually using >10 atm of pressure) (Fig. 4).[36]

In the current era of TCPVR, the most widely used valves in patients with CHD are the Melody valve and Edwards Sapien valve (Fig. 5). The Melody valve is a bovine jugular vein cuff and valve sewn onto a platinum iridium stent frame. The valve sizes range from 18 to 22 mm but the valve functions well at a greater range of implant diameters (12–24 mm).[35] The valve is hand mounted onto a covered balloon in a balloon delivery system (Ensemble), which is a 22F catheter diameter and is delivered via the femoral or jugular vein. The large size of the delivery system is not problematic in patients with ACHD but limits the use of this system in infants and young children in whom hybrid placement is considered. The Melody valve has been used for pulmonary stenosis and regurgitation, and at the time of this publication, had exceeded 10,000 implants in the United States.[35]

The Edwards Sapien valve is now in the third generation (the first generation is no longer commercially available). The second generation Sapien XT is Food and Drug Administration approved for use in dysfunctional conduits and the Sapien S3 is currently in an ongoing clinical trial evaluating its effectiveness for TCPVR in both conduits and bioprosthetic valves (COMPASSION S3 Clinical Trial NCT02744677). Both the XT and S3 are made of bovine pericardial tissue hand sewn onto a cobalt chromium stent platform with the addition of an expanded polytetrafluoroethylene cuff or skirt on the S3 model around the base. The Sapien valves range in size from 20 to 29 mm outer diameters and are deployed through an expandable sheath design. The larger diameter of the Sapien valves allows for the treatment of conduits, bioprostheses, and native RVOTs that exceed 24 mm in diameter and therefore cannot be treated with the Melody valve.

TECHNIQUE AND PERFORMANCE

Both the Melody and Sapien valves result in hemodynamic improvements, including reduction in stenosis and resolution of pulmonary regurgitation in most patients, with patients possessing predominant stenosis showing improved cardiorespiratory performance.[24,25,35,38] Procedural mortality and morbidity are low and comparable with surgical pulmonary valve replacement. Although the performance of both of these valves is excellent in the short term, on-going study is required to look at their long-term results.[38–40] Data are lacking on the long-term performance of the Sapien valve; however, the Melody valve 5-year outcomes are favorable with 76% of patients not requiring reintervention.[38] Surgical or transcatheter reintervention is most likely in those that experience infective endocarditis or valve stent frame fracture following TCPVR. The incidence of endocarditis of transcatheter valves has been found to be 3% to 25% and has been associated with several factors including abrupt cessation of antiplatelet therapy, male gender, failure to use spontaneous bacterial endocarditis prophylaxis, poor dental hygiene, untreated skin infections, prior episodes of endocarditis, stenotic conduits, residual stenosis post-TCPVR, and nail biting.[33]

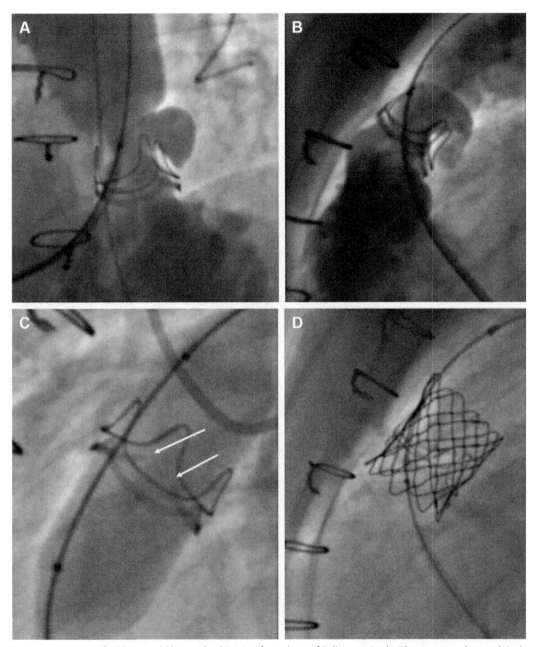

Fig. 4. Angiogram of a 12-year-old boy with a history of tetralogy of Fallot repaired with a transannular patch in the newborn period who later had a pulmonary valve replaced surgically with a 19-mm Magna Ease valve (Edwards Lifesciences, Irvine, CA) (*A, B*). Balloon sizing demonstrated a narrowed waist to 13.5 mm, which was believed to be much too small for this patient, who already had systemic right ventricular pressures and 40 mm Hg across the valve. Intentional annular fracture was achieved with a 20 mm VIDA balloon at 20 atm and could be seen on fluoroscopy during inflation (*arrows*) and felt by the practitioner (*C*). The patient then had a Melody valve placed on a 20-mm Ensemble, postdilated to 22 mm, with improvement in hemodynamics (*D*).

Although there are minimal data comparing the rate of incidence of endocarditis between the Melody and Sapien valves, there is a growing body of data suggesting a higher rate of incidence of endocarditis in bovine jugular tissues and an increased likelihood of bacterial adhesion to jugular venous material when compared with other valvular tissue.[32]

Stent fracture has been noted to be a problem with the Melody valve, especially when prestenting is not performed within conduits or native RVOTs. Prestenting does not seem to

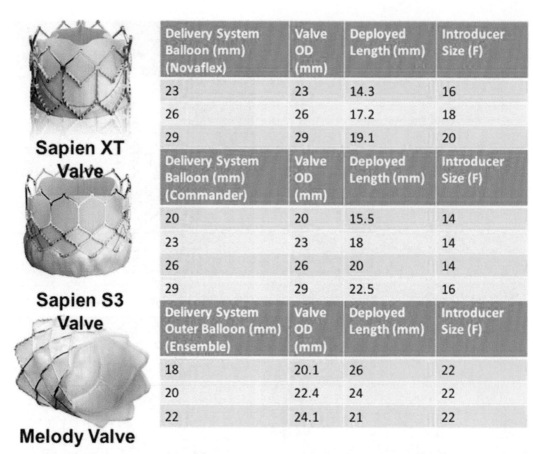

Delivery System Balloon (mm) (Novaflex)	Valve OD (mm)	Deployed Length (mm)	Introducer Size (F)
23	23	14.3	16
26	26	17.2	18
29	29	19.1	20
Delivery System Balloon (mm) (Commander)	Valve OD (mm)	Deployed Length (mm)	Introducer Size (F)
20	20	15.5	14
23	23	18	14
26	26	20	14
29	29	22.5	16
Delivery System Outer Balloon (mm) (Ensemble)	Valve OD (mm)	Deployed Length (mm)	Introducer Size (F)
18	20.1	26	22
20	22.4	24	22
22	24.1	21	22

Fig. 5. Figure highlighting some of the differences in the measured lengths, final outer diameter size, and French catheter size of the introducer. The 22-mm Melody valve is the longest valve, and the 23-mm Sapien XT the shortest. The Sapien valves are able to treat landing zones up to 29 mm, whereas the Melody valve halts at 24 mm. OD, outer diameter. (*Courtesy of* [Melody valve] Medtronic, Inc, Minneapolis, MN, with permission; and [Sapien XT] Edwards Lifesciences, Inc, Irvine, CA, with permission.)

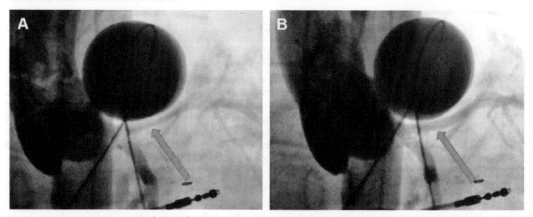

Fig. 6. Coronary compression of the left anterior descending (*blue arrows*) at its bifurcation at full inflation of the balloon catheter in the pulmonary artery (*A*), and re-establishment of flow when the balloon begins to deflate (*B*) in a patient undergoing an evaluation for possible transcatheter pulmonary valve replacement. This is a positive test of coronary compression and this patient did not have a transcatheter pulmonary valve replacement.

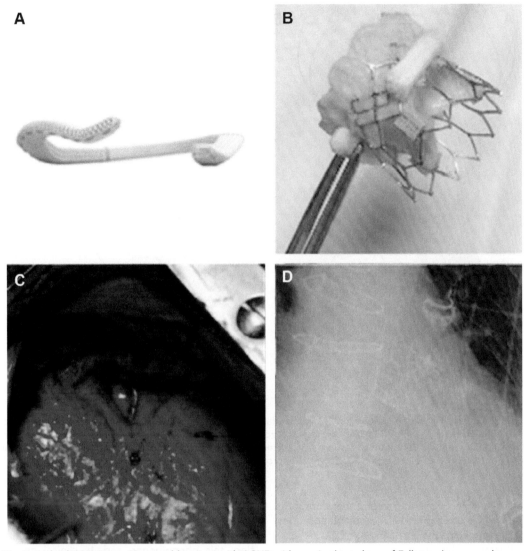

Fig. 7. Hybrid TCPVR in a 68-year-old patient with ACHD with repaired tetralogy of Fallot and severe pulmonary regurgitation. The patient presented with decompensated right ventricular failure, severely depressed right ventricular systolic function, and severe pulmonary regurgitation. He had undergone pulmonary valvectomy in childhood and had suffered from severe pulmonary regurgitation for six decades. Additionally, he suffered from renal dysfunction and congestive hepatopathy. He was deemed an extremely high-risk surgical candidate. The RVOT/main pulmonary artery measured 33 mm in minimum diameter; therefore, a hybrid TCPVR procedure was planned. (*A*) An Edwards 28-mm tricuspid annuloplasty physio band was used. (*B*) Initially this was bench tested with a 29-mm S3 valve implanted ex vivo. (*C*) In vivo implantation of the band via a median sternotomy. (*D*) Chest radiograph (anteroposterior view) following implantation of a 29-mm Sapien S3 within the banded pulmonary artery. ([*A*] *Courtesy of* Edwards Lifesciences Inc, Irvine, CA; with permission.)

be necessary in bioprosthetic valves given the presence of a metallic or plastic ring within which the stent platform is protected from compressive forces.[41] The platinum-iridium frame of the Melody valve may not be able to resist the compressive forces on it through the cardiac cycle, and especially when placed in close proximity to the sternum.[41] In the absence of prestenting of conduits and native RVOTs the stent fracture rate may exceed 25%; however, most stent fractures are type 1 wherein there remains structural integrity. The current practice standard is to prestent before Melody valve placement in conduits and native RVOTs, which has led to a dramatic decrease in Melody valve fracture rate (<5%).[38,41] The Sapien valve's cobalt chromium stent frame is significantly more durable, able to withstand high compressive

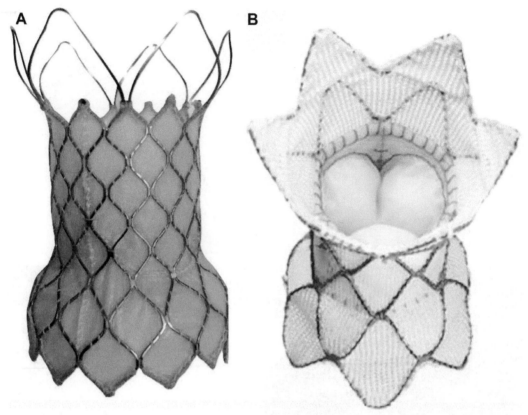

Fig. 8. The Venus P valve (riginal iteration) (*A*) and the Harmony valve (*B*) are two valves designed to applications to treat large-diameter native RVOTs. ([A] *Courtesy of* MedTech, Hongzhou, China; with permission; and *Data from* Jones MI, Qureshi SA. Recent advances in transcatheter management of pulmonary regurgitation after surgical repair of tetralogy of Fallot [version 1; referees: 3 approved]. F1000Res 2018;7. [pii:F1000 Faculty Rev-679].)

forces, and not prone to fracture; therefore, presenting before Sapien valve implantation does not seem necessary.[40,42]

It is imperative to evaluate for coronary arterial compression before valve implantation because coronary compression can occur in approximately 6% of patients.[43,44] Compression testing is performed by inflating a balloon with comparable size to the final diameter of the valve and stent to be delivered while simultaneously conducting coronary angiography either through selective coronary angiography, or through an aortic root angiogram (**Fig. 6**). Coronary artery compression is considered an absolute contraindication to percutaneous valve implantation.[44] High-risk substrates for coronary artery compression include those with anomalous coronary arterial anatomy and patients with surgically reimplanted coronary arteries.[43,44] More recently, the presence of aortic compression has been appreciated, wherein distortion of the aortic root results in aortic regurgitation during inflation of a sizing balloon

in the RVOT. This finding is in the context of an unpressurized aortic root because of the lack of forward cardiac output during balloon inflation; this phenomenon and its clinical consequences requires further study.[45]

The treatment of large-diameter (>30 mm) native RVOTs is especially challenging given that the largest commercially available balloon expandable TCPVR platforms are the 29-mm Sapien XT or Sapien 3 valves. The 29-mm Sapien 3 valve is expanded beyond its nominal diameter by overinflation with an additional 2 to 10 mL of volume with an eventual maximal outer diameter of 31 mm but this is not widely performed and one must consider the risk of compression of adjacent structures, valve embolization, and valvular or paravalvular regurgitation when the valve is overexpanded to this diameter in a native noncalcified. Hybrid surgical plication of the PA is considered via a sternotomy or thoracotomy to establish a "landing zone" for TCPVR.[46] The valve may then be deployed directly via the inferior wall of the RV or in the usual transvenous fashion (**Fig. 7**). The Venus P Valve (MedTech, Hongzhou, China) and the Harmony valve (Medtronic) are self-expanding covered hourglass-shaped RVOT reducer platforms with the valve in the central waist (**Fig. 8**). The Venus P valve has been safely implanted and early data have demonstrated improvement in hemodynamics and RV volume, whereas early feasibility studies of the Harmony valve showed improved hemodynamics, and only mild pulmonary regurgitation 1 year after implantation.[47–49] The Harmony valve is currently in a phase III multicenter clinical trial in the United States (The Medtronic Harmony TPV Clinical Trial NCT02979587). Edwards Lifesciences has developed a self-expanding RVOT reducer that does not house a valve platform, the Alterra adaptive RVOT reducer. The Sapien-3 29-mm valve is subsequently implanted within the Alterra RVOT reducer. These devices targeting reducing the RVOT are discussed in detail elsewhere in this issue.

SUMMARY

TCPVR in patients with dysfunctional RVOTs is feasible, safe, and efficacious. Multiple surgical pulmonary valve interventions are associated with higher risks of heart failure and arrhythmias in these patients as they grow older; therefore, nonsurgical techniques for pulmonary valve replacement are favored in this population. Commercially available platforms include the balloon expandable Melody and Sapien family of valves. The Melody valve is Food and Drug Administration approved for use in dysfunctional conduits and bioprosthetic valves, whereas the Sapien valve is approved for use in dysfunctional conduits. However, the Sapien valve is also widely used in large bioprosthetic valves and native RVOTs given the larger valve diameters available. Coronary arterial and aortic root compression should be considered before valve implantation. Valve stent fracture and infective endocarditis are long-term considerations following TCPVR. Very large native RVOTs (>30 mm) represent a challenging subset that may require hybrid surgical plication before balloon-expandable valve implantation. Several self-expanding platforms are currently being tested to address patients with large native RVOTs and predominantly severe regurgitation.

REFERENCES

1. Mandalenakis Z, Rosengren A, Skoglund K, et al. Survivorship in children and young adults with congenital heart disease in Sweden. JAMA Intern Med 2017;177(2):224–30.

2. Moons P, Bovijn L, Budts W, et al. Temporal trends in survival to adulthood among patients born with congenital heart disease from 1970 to 1992 in Belgium. Circulation 2010;122(22):2264–72.

3. Jilaihawi H, Kashif M, Fontana G, et al. Cross-sectional computed tomographic assessment improves accuracy of aortic annular sizing for transcatheter aortic valve replacement and reduces the incidence of paravalvular aortic regurgitation. J Am Coll Cardiol 2012;59(14):1275–86.

4. Georges JL, Belle L, Ricard C, et al, RAY'ACT Investigators. Patient exposure to X-rays during coronary angiography and percutaneous transluminal coronary intervention: results of a multicenter national survey. Catheter Cardiovasc Interv 2014;83(5):729–38.

5. Papadopoulou DI, Yakoumakis EN, Makri TK, et al. Assessment of patient radiation doses during transcatheter closure of ventricular and atrial septal defects with Amplatzer devices. Catheter Cardiovasc Interv 2005;65(3):434–41.

6. Glatz AC, Purrington KS, Klinger A, et al. Cumulative exposure to medical radiation for children requiring surgery for congenital heart disease. J Pediatr 2014;164(4):789–94.e10.

7. Frigiola A, Giamberti A, Chessa M, et al. Right ventricular restoration during pulmonary valve implantation in adults with congenital heart disease. Eur J Cardiothorac Surg 2006;29:S279–85.

8. Geva T. Repaired tetralogy of Fallot: the roles of cardiovascular magnetic resonance in evaluating pathophysiology and for pulmonary valve replacement decision support. J Cardiovasc Magn Reson 2011;13:9–32.

9. Kiraly L, Tofeig M, Jha NK, et al. Three-dimensional printed prototypes refine the anatomy of post-modified Norwood-1 complex aortic arch obstruction and allow presurgical simulation of the repair. Interact Cardiovasc Thorac Surg 2016;22:238–40.

10. Yoo SJ, Thabit O, Kim EK, et al. 3D printing in medicine of congenital heart diseases. 3D Print Med 2016;2:3–15.

11. Hoang D, Perrault D, Stevanovic M, et al. Surgical applications of three-dimensional printing: a review of the current literature & how to get started. Ann Transl Med 2016;4:456.

12. Schmauss D, Haeberle S, Hagl C, et al. Three-dimensional printing in cardiac surgery and interventional cardiology: a single-centre experience. Eur J Cardiothorac Surg 2015;47:1044–52.

13. Awad SM, Masood SA, Gonzalez I, et al. The use of intracardiac echocardiography during percutaneous pulmonary valve replacement. Pediatr Cardiol 2015;36:76.

14. Baumgartner H, Hung J, Bermejo J, et al. Echocardiographic assessment of valve stenosis: EAE/ASE

recommendations for clinical practice. J Am Soc Echocardiogr 2009;22:1.

15. Bonhoeffer P, Boudjemline Y, Saliba Z, et al. Percutaneous replacement of pulmonary valve in a right-ventricle to pulmonary artery prosthetic conduit with valve dysfunction. Lancet 2000;356:1403–5.

16. Ferraz Cavalcanti PE, Sá MP, Santos CA, et al. Pulmonary valve replacement after operative repair of tetralogy of Fallot: metaanalysis and meta-regression of 3,118 patients from 48 studies. J Am Coll Cardiol 2013;62:2227–43.

17. Gillespie MJ, Rome JJ, Levi DS, et al. Melody valve implant within failed bioprosthetic valves in the pulmonary position: a multicenter experience. Circ Cardiovasc Interv 2012;5:862–70.

18. Cribier A, Eltchaninoff H, Bash A, et al. Percutaneous transcatheter implantation of an aortic valve prosthesis for calcific aortic stenosis: first human case description. Circulation 2002;106:3006—8.

19. Davies H. Catheter-mounted valve for temporary relief of aortic insufficiency. Lancet 1965;285:250.

20. Lee C, Kim YM, Lee CH, et al. Outcomes of pulmonary valve replacement in 170 patients with chronic pulmonary regurgitation after relief of right ventricular outflow tract obstruction: implications for optimal timing of pulmonary valve replacement. J Am Coll Cardiol 2012;60:1005–14.

21. Borik S, Crean A, Horlick E, et al. Percutaneous pulmonary valve implantation: 5 years of follow-up: does age influence outcomes? Circ Cardiovasc Interv 2015;8:e001745.

22. Ong K, Boone R, Gao M, et al. Right ventricle to pulmonary artery conduit reoperations in patients with tetralogy of Fallot of pulmonary atresia associated with ventricular septal defect. Am J Cardiol 2013;111:1638–43.

23. Labombarda F, Hamilton R, Shohoudi A, et al. Increasing prevalence of atrial fibrillation and permanent atrial arrhythmias in congenital heart disease. J Am Coll Cardiol 2017;70:857–65.

24. Lurz P, Riede FT, Taylor AM, et al. Impact of percutaneous pulmonary valve implantation for right ventricular outflow tract dysfunction on exercise recovery kinetics. Int J Cardiol 2014;177:276–80.

25. Batra AS, McElhinney DB, Wang W, et al. Cardiopulmonary exercise function among patients undergoing transcatheter pulmonary valve implantation in the US Melody valve investigational trial. Am Heart J 2012;163:280–7.

26. Knauth AL, Gauvreau K, Powell AJ, et al. Ventricular size and function assessed by cardiac MRI predict major adverse clinical outcomes late after tetralogy of Fallot repair. Heart 2008;94:211–6.

27. Stark J, Bull C, Stajevic M, et al. LevalFate of sub-pulmonary homograft conduits: determinants of late homograft failure. J Thorac Cardiovasc Surg 1998;115:506–14 [discussion: 514–6].

28. Morray BH, McElhinney DB, Boudjemline Y, et al. Multicentre experience evaluating transcatheter pulmonary valve replacement in bovine jugular vein (Contegra) right ventricle to pulmonary artery conduits. Circ Cardiovasc Interv 2017;10:e004914.

29. Butera G, Milanesi O, Spadoni I, et al. Melody transcatheter pulmonary valve implantation. Results from the registry of the Italian Society of Pediatric Cardiology. Catheter Cardiovasc Interv 2013; 81:310–6.

30. Cheatham SL, Holzer RJ, Chisolm JL, et al. The Medtronic Melody® transcatheter pulmonary valve implanted at 24-mm diameter—it works. Catheter Cardiovasc Interv 2013;82:816–23.

31. Sharma A, Cote AT, Hosking KC, et al. A systematic review of infective endocarditis in patients with bovine jugular vein valves compared with other valve types. JACC Cardiovasc Interv 2017;10(14): 1449–58.

32. Jalal Z, Galmiche L, Lebeaux D, et al. Selective propensity of bovine jugular vein material to bacterial adhesions: an in-vitro study. Int J Cardiol 2015; 198:201–5.

33. Lluri G, Levi DS, Miller E. Incidence and outcome of infective endocarditis following percutaneous versus surgical pulmonary valve replacement. Catheter Cardiovasc Interv 2017. https://doi.org/10. 1002/ccd.27312.

34. Belli E, Salihoğlu E, Leobon B, et al. The performance of Hancock porcine-valved Dacron conduit for right ventricular outflow tract reconstruction. Ann Thorac Surg 2010;89(1):152–7.

35. Cheatham JP, Hellenbrand WE, Zahn EM, et al. Clinical and hemodynamic outcomes up to 7 years after transcatheter pulmonary valve replacement in the US Melody valve investigational device exemption trial. Circulation 2015;131:1960–70.

36. Tanase D, Grohmann J, Schubert S, et al. Cracking the ring of Edwards Perimount bioprosthesis with ultrahigh pressure balloons prior to transcatheter valve in valve implantation. Int J Cardiol 2014;176: 1048–9.

37. Si MS. Open Melody implant in a vascular graft—An alternative to the bioprosthetic valve? J Thorac Cardiovasc Surg 2018;155(2):742–74.

38. McElhinney DB, Hellenbrand WE, Zahn EM, et al. Short- and medium-term outcomes after transcatheter pulmonary valve placement in the expanded multicenter US Melody valve trial. Circulation 2010;122(5):507–16.

39. Levi DS, Sinha S, Salem MM, et al. Transcatheter native pulmonary valve and tricuspid valve replacement with the Sapien XT: initial experience and development of a new delivery platform. Catheter Cardiovasc Interv 2016;88(3):434–43.

40. Ghobrial J, Levi DS, Aboulhosn J. Native right ventricular outflow tract transcatheter pulmonary valve

replacement without pre-stenting. JACC Cardiovasc Interv 2018;11(6):e41–4.

41. Cardoso R, Ansari M, Garcia D, et al. Prestenting for prevention of Melody valve stent fractures: a systematic review and metaanalysis. Catheter Cardiovasc Interv 2016;87:534–9. JACC Cardiovasc Interv 2017;10(14):1449–58.

42. Tzamtzis S, Viquerat J, Yap J, et al. BurriesciNumerical analysis of the radial force produced by the Medtronic-CoreValve and Edwards-SAPIEN after transcatheter aortic valve implantation (TAVR). Med Eng Phys 2013;35:125–30.

43. Fraisse A, Assaidi A, Mauri L, et al. Coronary artery compression during intention to treat right ventricle outflow with percutaneous pulmonary valve implantation: incidence, diagnosis, and outcome. Catheter Cardiovasc Interv 2014;83:E260–8.

44. Morray BH, McElhinney DB, Cheatham JP, et al. Risk of coronary artery compression among patients referred for transcatheter pulmonary valve implantation: a multicenter experience. Circ Cardiovasc Interv 2013;6:535–42.

45. Lindsay I, Aboulhosn J, Salem M3, et al. Aortic root compression during transcatheter pulmonary valve replacement. Catheter Cardiovasc Interv 2016; 88(5):814–21.

46. Rapetto F, Kenny D, Caputo M. Editorial: the developments of hybrid surgical strategies for congenital heart disease. Front Surg 2017;4:55.

47. Cao QL, Kenny D, Zhou D, et al. Early clinical experience with a novel self-expanding percutaneous stent-valve in the native right ventricular out ow tract. Catheter Cardiovasc Interv 2014;84: 1131–7.

48. Bergersen L, Benson LN, Gillespie MJ, et al. Harmony feasibility trial: acute and short-term outcomes with a self-expanding transcatheter pulmonary valve. JACC Cardiovasc Interv 2017;10: 1763–73.

49. Jones MI, Qureshi SA. Recent advances in transcatheter management of pulmonary regurgitation after surgical repair of tetralogy of Fallot [version 1; referees: 3 approved]. F1000Res 2018;7 [pii: F1000 Faculty Rev-679].

Self-Expanding Pulmonary Valves for Large Diameter Right Ventricular Outflow Tracts

Evan Michael Zahn, MD

KEYWORDS

- Pulmonary regurgitation • Native right ventricular outflow tract • Transcatheter pulmonary valve

KEY POINTS

- The "native" right ventricular outflow tract presents unique challenges in terms of designing a transcatheter pulmonary valve.
- Several designs are currently being evaluated and are in the early stages of development and testing.
- With further experience and technical modifications, transcatheter pulmonary valve placement in the native right ventricular outflow tract will soon be a reality.

INTRODUCTION

Congenital heart defects that involve obstruction to the right ventricular outflow tract (RVOT) are common and include tetralogy of Fallot, pulmonary valve stenosis, and pulmonary atresia. Tetralogy of Fallot is the most common cyanotic heart disease, occurring in approximately 1 in 2518 births in the United Sates.[1] Surgical repair of these lesions typically involves early relief of RVOT obstruction, which may include pulmonary valvotomy or valvectomy, RVOT muscular resection, and, in the case of tetralogy of Fallot, a transannular patch. These operations nearly universally result in significant pulmonary insufficiency, which, although well-tolerated in childhood, often results in long-term sequelae such as right ventricular dilation and dysfunction, arrhythmia, limited exercise capacity, right heart failure, and sudden death.[2–7] Surgical pulmonary valve replacement is a time-tested and well-tolerated operation with acceptable morbidity, mortality, and long-term outcomes.[8–11] That being said, these operations carry with them the physical and psychological

discomfort associated with any repeat open heart surgical procedure and in general patients wish to avoid them. Transcatheter pulmonary valve replacement (TPVR), first described by Bonhoeffer and associates[12] nearly 20 years ago, has revolutionized treatment of RVOT dysfunction, particularly in patients with previously placed and subsequently failed surgical valves such as right ventricular–pulmonary artery conduits and bioprosthetic valves.[13,14] Currently approved devices for TPVR in the United States include the Melody transcatheter pulmonary valve (Medtronic, Minneapolis, MN) and the Edwards SAPIEN XT™ valve (Edwards Life Science, Irvine, CA), both of which are balloon-expandable stent-mounted valves approved for treatment of dysfunctional conduits and bioprosthetic valves in the pulmonic position. By their design, neither valve is ideally suited for treatment of the large, dilated, so-called native RVOT, typically encountered after a transannular patch repair or pulmonary valvotomy/valvectomy. While several innovative methods have been developed to successfully treat this patient population with currently available balloon

Disclosure Statement: Edwards Life Sciences—consult, proctor, National PI Alterra/S3 study. Medtronic—proctor, consultant; Med-Zenith Medical Scientific Co.—consultant.

Guerin Family Congenital Heart Program, Cedars Sinai Medical Center, 127 South San Vicente Boulevard, Los Angeles, CA 90048, USA

E-mail address: evan.zahn@cshs.org

expandable valves (particularly the larger diameter SAPIEN valves) the vast majority of these patients continue to require surgery secondary to a lack of a suitable device designed for this specific population.[15–20]

In this article, we review the current status of a new generation of self-expanding valves currently being developed for TPVR use in so-called native, large diameter RVOTs.

CHALLENGES IN DEVELOPING A SUITABLE DEVICE

After surgical (eg, transannular patch) or transcatheter treatment of RVOT obstruction (eg, balloon pulmonary valvuloplasty) in infancy, a number of changes occur within the RVOT and main pulmonary artery over time that pose significant engineering challenges to designing a single transcatheter device, particularly a balloon-expandable one, for this complex population.

Challenge 1: Interpatient Variability

Schievano and colleagues[21] demonstrated using cardiac MRI and 3-dimensional volume analysis the wide interpatient variability in RVOT morphology after common RVOT interventions (Fig. 1). Although these investigators were able to divide 83 patient's RVOT anatomies into 5

visually identifiable patterns, there continued to be wide variability within each category. Furthermore, no direct correlation was found between surgical history or underlying diagnosis and subsequent RVOT morphologic classification confirming the unpredictability and wide interpatient variability encountered within this population.

Challenge 2: Marked Variability in Right Ventricular Outflow Tract Dimensions Throughout the Cardiac Cycle

Using 4-dimensional computed tomography scanning, these same investigators[20] demonstrated that within an individual patient there is marked anatomic variability, which occurs within the RVOT throughout the cardiac cycle in terms of cross-sectional areas, perimeters, and maximum and minimum diameters (Fig. 2). Notably, RVOT diameters where transcatheter valves could potentially be placed, varied by more than 50% throughout the cardiac cycle. Additionally, the authors noted that there was tremendous axial deformation (shortening and lengthening) of the RVOT (as much as 80%) during various portions of the cardiac cycle, adding to the complexity of these dynamic structures.

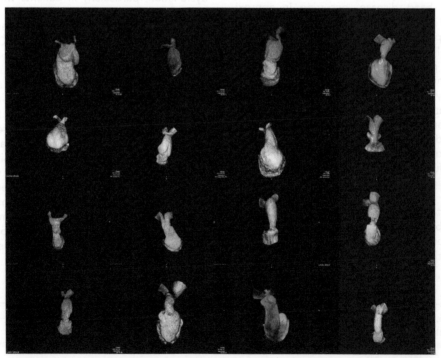

Fig. 1. Sixteen consecutively obtained images of patients with postoperative right ventricular outflow tract disease using 3-dimensional reconstructed images obtained with rotational angiography. Note the remarkable interpatient variability.

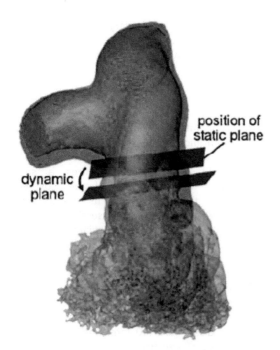

position of
static plane

dynamic
plane

Fig. 2. Superimposed computed tomography acquired systolic (*red*) and diastolic (*blue*) volumes of a patient with a large patched right ventricular outflow tract showing the marked variability in the cross-sectional area and supraannular plane and length, which occurs during the cardiac cycle.

Challenge 3: Irregular Shape

Current balloon-expandable valves were designed to be placed within relatively circular or cylindrical locations such as conduits, bioprosthetic valves, or the aortic annulus (in the case of Sapien valves). The irregular geometric configuration of the RVOT after surgical reconstruction, further distorted by years of pulmonary insufficiency, poses a significant engineering challenge.

Challenge 4: Large Size and Unpredictable Compliance

The sheer diameter, perimeter, and cross-sectional areas of the reconstructed, dilated RVOT coupled with the unpredictable compliance of these structures make designing a simple balloon-expandable valve for this location daunting.

These challenges have resulted in the development of a number of novel designs currently undergoing clinical evaluation for this unique application. All of these devices share in common the use of self-expanding memory alloys in their frame design. These alloys offer the potential to be versatile in design and construction, thereby offering the possibility of adaptation to the widely variable geometry of the reconstructed/ regurgitant RVOT. Additionally, these materials

have proven biocompatibility and possess the potential to undergo large, reversible deformations as seen throughout the cardiac cycle in this location, offering the possibility of frame fracture resistance. Currently, 3 self-expanding transcatheter pulmonary valves are in clinical trials and are described herein.

CURRENT SELF-EXPANDING VALVES FOR THE LARGE RIGHT VENTRICULAR OUTFLOW TRACT

Medtronic Harmony Transcatheter Pulmonary Valve

In 2010, the group at Great Ormond Street led by Phillip Bonhoeffer published the first percutaneous human implant of a self-expanding custom designed pulmonary valve for treatment of pulmonary regurgitation in 42-year-old man with a large dilated outflow tract.[22] This original design ultimately evolved into the Harmony Transcatheter Pulmonary Valve. Perhaps more important, the preimplant imaging evaluation of this patient, which involved the use of 4-dimensional computed tomography data to create computational and rapid prototyping models of the RVOT have become an important mainstay for current patient screening for these new devices.[23,24] The Harmony valve is composed of a porcine pericardial tissue valve mounted within a covered nitinol self-expanding frame (**Fig. 3**).[25] The current device

A

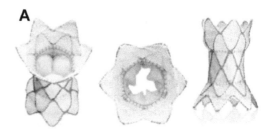

B

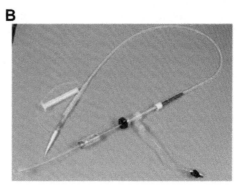

Fig. 3. Medtronic Harmony Transcatheter Pulmonary Valve (*A*) and its accompanying delivery system (*B*). (*Courtesy of* Medtronic, Inc, Minneapolis, MN; with permission.)

comes in 1 size that has a length of 55 mm and an asymmetrical design with the following outer diameters: pulmonary outflow of 34 mm, valved section of 23.5 mm, and inflow of 42 mm. The valve is treated with an alpha amino oleic acid antimineralization process to mitigate leaflet calcification and is sterilized with a 0.2% glutaraldehyde sterilant. The delivery system is 25 F with a coil loading system and integrated sheath. The valve is collapsed for loading with a plastic funnel and, once in the desired location, the valve is advanced into position over a stiff Lunderquist guidewire placed in the left pulmonary artery and deployed by retraction of the outer sheath. Deployment of the valve begins in the proximal left pulmonary artery, gradually exposing each strut until the valve is fully deployed in the main pulmonary artery. The most proximal strut is deployed into the distal RVOT and, once fully unsheathed, the valve is released from the delivery system by rotating the delivery handle, allowing the coil loading system to release the frame.

Results of an early US feasibility study have recently been published.[25] The device was successfully deployed in 20 of 21 catheterized patients. In short-term follow-up, 2 patients required surgical device removal (1 early distal migration within 24 hours and 1 proximal type II stent fracture resulting in an obstruction). Of the remaining 18 patients available for the 6-month evaluation, overall device integrity and functionality seemed to be well-maintained. All had persistent relief of clinically relevant pulmonary regurgitation and the RVOT mean gradient for the group seemed to remain stable at 15 ± 6 mm Hg. There were, however, 2 cases of mild paravalvar leak and a total of 3 patients who developed asymptomatic type I frame fracture. The authors concluded that, "The early clinical outcomes of the Harmony TPV demonstrate promising device performance and preservation of stent integrity in the majority of cases." However, importantly, they also noted that, "The results of the Harmony TPV study will be analyzed for product improvement and development of additional sizes to address the broad range of RVOT anatomies and of ways to maintain or improve device integrity." This final comment was based in part on the fact that the initial 21 catheterized patients were drawn from an initial cohort of 66 consented patients, 45 who were deemed to have inappropriate anatomy for this design. Although the initial Harmony valve has played an important role in the early evolution of this technology for patients with large and dilated RVOT, including the refinement of detailed screening methodology for this population, it will likely undergo significant redesign and expansion of available sizes before it becomes a clinical mainstay for this population.

The Venus P-Valve

As of this writing, the Venus P-Valve (Venus MedTech, Hangzhou, China) has been the most widely implanted self-expanding TPV in the world with more than 200 implants to date (Shakeel Quereshi, MD, personal communication, 2018). This device features a self-expandable nitinol support frame covered throughout the majority of its length with porcine pericardial tissue possessing an integrated trileaflet porcine pericardial tissue valve (Fig. 4). The distal outflow row of cells is left uncovered to allow for unobstructed branch pulmonary artery flow. The device is flared at the proximal and distal ends (both 10 mm larger in diameter than the central valve housing) with the proximal flare being 2 mm longer (12 mm) than the distal flare (10 mm) and comes in a wide variety of size from valve housing diameters between 18 and 36 mm (in 2-mm increments) and lengths between 20 and 35 mm (in 5-mm increments). There are 3 sets of radiopaque marker bands identifying the distal flare, valve position, and proximal flare. The delivery system consists of a 16 F 100-cm-long shaft catheter with a 20 F to 22 F capsule and a handle rotating mechanism for controlled deployment of the valve. The valved stent is crimped and loaded onto the delivery system under sterile cold saline solution, which helps to decrease the memory property of nitinol. The delivery system is advanced through a 22 F to 24 F sheath. Although a worldwide trial is currently ongoing, currently published reports contain just a few patients. In 2014, Cao and colleagues[26] published the first report of 5 adult congenital patients (median weight, 55 kgs), who were successfully implanted in China with this device. All were symptomatic with severe pulmonary insufficiency and dilated right ventricles. Reported follow-up was short (mean, 3.4 ± 2.5 months), but the results are encouraging, with no patient having more than trivial pulmonary insufficiency, no evidence for RVOT obstruction, and a trend toward diminished right ventricular volumes. More recently, Garay and colleagues[27] have published a series of 10 symptomatic patients (New York Heart Association functional class II and III) after patients with tetralogy of Fallot, who all underwent successful valve implantation with no reported procedural complications. Six-month follow-up data showed marked improvements in pulmonary regurgitant fraction

A

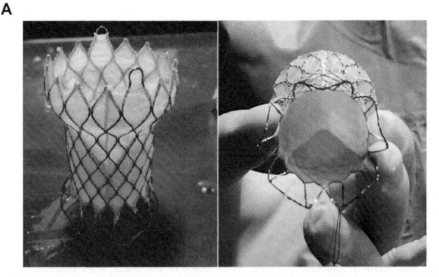

B

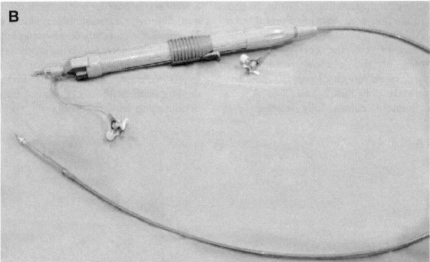

Fig. 4. The Venus P Valve. (A) The distal outflow portion is uncovered while the proximal end is marked by the 2 hooks used to attach the device to the delivery system (B). (*Courtesy of* Venus MedTech, Shanghai, China; with permission.)

by both echocardiography and MRI with all patients reported to be New York Heart Association functional class I at 12 months. Three complications have been reported to date in the literature.[28] Two of these involved incomplete expansion of the valve frame during delivery, both of which were successfully treated with balloon expansion of the valve; however, one of these resulted in leaflet dysfunction and severe pulmonary regurgitation. The other complication described involved proximal device migration occurring during delivery system withdrawal, resulting in mild paravalve leak and significant tricuspid valve regurgitation.

A much larger multisite, multinational trial is currently ongoing and should provide greater insight into the ultimate place this valve will have in the treatment of this population.

The Alterra Adaptive Prestent/Sapien S3

The Alterra™ Adaptive Prestent (Edwards Lifesciences, Irvine, CA) is designed to be used as a docking adaptor for the 29-mm SAPIEN 3™ transcatheter heart valve within the RVOT. This concept and design differs from both the Harmony and Venus P valves in that it involves initial placement of the Alterra prestent to reshape the RVOT, followed (at the same procedure or at a later separate procedure) by placement of a SAPIEN S3 valve within the stent.

It is composed of a self-expanding, radiopaque, nitinol frame assembly and polyethylene terephthalate fabric covering and has designated inflow and outflow ends (Fig. 5). The inflow section is identifiable by the presence of 2 triangular tabs that are attached to the delivery system and circumferential covering of all cells. The outflow section is distinguished by open cells designed to facilitate blood flow into the branch pulmonary arteries should the device need to extend into the orifice of one or both of these structures. The polyethylene terephthalate fabric is attached by sutures to the inside surface of the frame to create a seal at the inflow section. The device has a symmetric frame design with the inflow and outflow diameters equal to 40 mm and the central section is 27 mm to provide a rigid landing zone for a SAPIEN 3 valve (29 mm). Although the total unconstrained device length is 48 mm, the non–fabric-coated row of cells at the outflow results in a completely covered length of only 30 mm. The device currently only has 2 size. The Alterra Adaptive Prestent comes fully loaded in a

custom delivery system consisting of a handle, retractable outer shaft, inner delivery shaft (upon which the stent sits), prestent connector, and a tapered tip meant to facilitate tracking through the vasculature (see Fig. 5). The delivery handle consists of a single knob that ergonomically allows for a 1-handed, slow, controlled deployment and potential recapture and a flush port to flush the guidewire lumen (consistent with a 0.035″ guidewire). The entire system fits through a 16 F eSheath™ (Edwards Life Sciences, Irvine, CA). The device is advanced over a rigid guidewire into one of the branch pulmonary arteries (typically left) where deployment of the distal apices begins. Once the distal cells are partially deployed, the device is pulled back into the desired final deployment location and the remaining stent deployed. Following assessment of the result, a 29 mm SAPIEN 3 valve is advanced in to the midportion of the Alterra and deployed with simple balloon expansion. This device is currently undergoing initial evaluation within an early feasibility study in the United States.[28] Only a single case report has been published to date describing the first successful implant with a good procedural outcome and encouraging early follow-up.

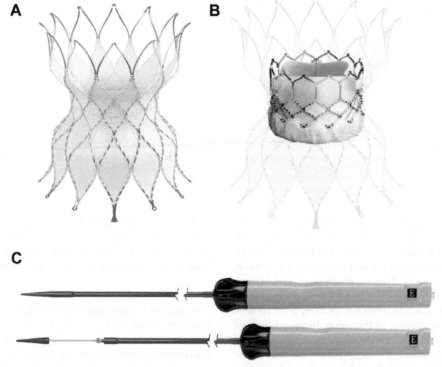

Fig. 5. The Alterra Adaptive Prestent shown alone (*A*) and with the Sapien S3 implanted within the designated landing zone (*B*). Note the symmetric design dimensions; however, the distal outflow is uncovered and the inflow section is covered and marked by 2 tabs used to attach the device to the delivery system (*C*). (*Courtesy of* Edwards Lifesciences, Irvine, CA; with permission.)

SUMMARY

It is clear that the complex and varied anatomy of the large native or patched RVOT presents quite a challenge in designing a suitable trans-catheter valve alternative. This is an exciting time as partnerships of clinicians, engineers, and corporate entities are collaborating around the world to design systems specifically to address these challenging patients. As experience grows and further refinements are made with the devices described herein and others still in development, there is little doubt that a viable catheter-based alternative (likely several) for TPVR in this population will soon be available as a practical clinical alternative to surgical valve replacement.

REFERENCES

1. Parker SE, Mai CT, Canfield MA, et al. Updated National Birth Prevalence estimates for selected birth defects in the United States, 2004–2006. Birth Defects Res A Clin Mol Teratol 2010;88:1008–16.
2. Bove EL, Byrum CJ, Thomas FD, et al. The influence of pulmonary insufficiency on ventricular function following repair of tetralogy of Fallot. Evaluation using radionuclide ventriculography. J Thorac Cardiovasc Surg 1983;85:691–6.
3. Niezen RA, Helbing WA, van der Wall EE, et al. Biventricular systolic function and mass studied 918.
4. Gatzoulis MA, Till JA, Somerville J, et al. Mechanoelectrical interaction in tetralogy of Fallot. QRS prolongation relates to right ventricular size and predicts malignant ventricular arrhythmia and sudden death. Circulation 1995;92:231–7.
5. Rowe SA, Zahka KG, Manolio TA, et al. Lung function and pulmonary regurgitation limit exercise capacity in postoperative tetralogy of Fallot. J Am Coll Cardiol 1991;17:461–6.
6. Kondo C, Nakazawa M, Kusakabe K, et al. Left ventricular dysfunction on exercise long-term after total repair of tetralogy of Fallot. Circulation 1995;92:II250–5.
7. Gatzoulis MA, Balaji S, Webber SA, et al. Risk factors for arrhythmia and sudden cardiac death late after repair of tetralogy of Fallot: a multicentre study. Lancet 2000;356:975–81.
8. Khanna AD, Hill KD, Pasquali SK, et al. Benchmark outcomes for pulmonary valve replacement using the society of thoracic surgeons databases. Ann Thorac Surg 2015;100:138–45.
9. Sabate Rotes A, Eidem BW, Connolly HM, et al. Long-term follow-up after pulmonary valve replacement in repaired tetralogy of Fallot. Am J Cardiol 2014;114:901–8.

10. Babu-Narayan SV, Diller GP, Gheta RR, et al. Clinical outcomes of surgical pulmonary valve replacement after repair of tetralogy of Fallot and potential prognostic value of preoperative cardiopulmonary exercise testing. Circulation 2014;129:18–27.
11. Ferraz Cavalcanti PE, Sa MP, Santos CA, et al. Pulmonary valve replacement after operative repair of tetralogy of Fallot: meta-analysis and meta-regression of 3,118 patients from 48 studies. J Am Coll Cardiol 2013;62:2227–43.
12. Bonhoeffer P, Boudjemline Y, Saliba Z, et al. Percutaneous replacement of pulmonary valve in a right-ventricle to pulmonary-artery prosthetic conduit with valve dysfunction. Lancet 2000;356:1403–5.
13. McElhinney DB, Hellenbrand WE, Zahn EM, et al. Short- and medium-term outcomes after transcatheter pulmonary valve placement in the expanded multicenter US melody valve trial. Circulation 2010;122(5):507–16.
14. Cheatham JP, Hellenbrand WE, Zahn EM, et al. Clinical and hemodynamic outcomes up to 7 years after transcatheter pulmonary valve replacement in the US melody valve investigational device exemption trial. Circulation 2015;131(22):1960–70.
15. Meadows JJ, Moore PM, Berman DP, et al. Use and performance of the Melody transcatheter pulmonary valve in native and postsurgical, nonconduit right ventricular outflow tracts. Circ Cardiovasc Interv 2014;7(3):374–80.
16. Malekzadeh-Milani S, Ladouceur M, Cohen S, et al. Results of transcatheter pulmonary valvulation in native or patched right ventricular outflow tracts. Arch Cardiovasc Dis 2014;107(11):592–8.
17. Guccione P, Milanesi O, Hijazi ZM, et al. Transcatheter pulmonary valve implantation in native pulmonary outflow tract using the Edwards SAPIEN™ transcatheter heart valve. Eur J Cardiothorac Surg 2012;41(5):1192–4.
18. Sosnowski C, Matella T, Fogg L, et al. Hybrid pulmonary artery plication followed by transcatheter pulmonary valve replacement: comparison with surgical PVR. Catheter Cardiovasc Interv 2016;88(5):804–10.
19. Phillips AB, Nevin P, Shah A, et al. Development of a novel hybrid strategy for transcatheter pulmonary valve placement in patients following transannular patch repair of tetralogy of fallot. Catheter Cardiovasc Interv 2016;87(3):403–10.
20. Schievano S, Capelli C, Young C, et al. Four-dimensional computed tomography: a method of assessing right ventricular outflow tract and pulmonary artery deformations throughout the cardiac cycle. Eur Radiol 2011;21(1):36–45.
21. Schievano S, Coats L, Migliavacca F, et al. Variations in right ventricular outflow tract morphology following repair of congenital heart disease:

implications for percutaneous pulmonary valve implantation. J Cardiovasc Magn Reson 2007;9(4): 687–95.

22. Schievano S, Taylor AM, Capelli C, et al. VFirst-in-man implantation of a novel percutaneous valve: a new approach to medical device development. EuroIntervention 2010;5(6):745–50.

23. Capelli C, Taylor AM, Migliavacca F, et al. Patient-specific reconstructed anatomies and computer simulations are fundamental for selecting medical device treatment: application to a new percutaneous pulmonary valve. Philos Trans A Math Phys Eng Sci 2010;368(1921):3027–38.

24. Gillespie MJ, Benson LN, Bergersen L, et al. Patient selection process for the harmony transcatheter pulmonary valve early feasibility study. Am J Cardiol 2017;120(8):1387–92.

25. Bergersen L, Benson LN, Gillespie MJ, et al. Harmony feasibility trial: acute and short-term outcomes with a self-expanding transcatheter pulmonary valve. JACC Cardiovasc Interv 2017;10(17):1763–73.

26. Cao QL, Kenny D, Zhou D, et al. Early clinical experience with a novel self-expanding percutaneous stent-valve in the native right ventricular outflow tract. Catheter Cardiovasc Interv 2014;84(7):1131–7.

27. Garay F, Pan X, Zhang YJ, et al. Early experience with the Venus p-valve for percutaneous pulmonary valve implantation in native outflow tract. Neth Heart J 2017;25(2):76–81.

28. Zahn EM, Chang JC, Amer D, et al. First human implant of the Alterra Adaptive Prestent[tm]: a new self expanding device designed to remodel the right ventricular outflow tract. Catheter Cardiovasc Interv 2018;91(6):1125–9.

Biodegradable Stents for Congenital Heart Disease

Tre R. Welch, PhD[a], Alan W. Nugent, MBBS, FRACP[b],
Surendranath R. Veeram Reddy, MD[c],*

KEYWORDS

- Biodegradable stents • Bioresorbable polymers • Biocorrodible metals
- Congenital heart disease • Pediatric stents • Poly-L-lactic-acid

KEY POINTS

- Patients with congenital heart disease will benefit the most from a biodegradable stent that will relieve the obstruction and eventually disappear allowing for normal future vessel growth.
- Infants and children born with congenital heart disease need larger diameter stents to treat obstructed blood vessels such as the aorta and pulmonary arteries.
- There are significant biomedical and engineering challenges related to decreasing collapse pressure and increasing elastic recoil with fabrication of larger diameter biodegradable stents.
- Current research is focused on identifying optimal biodegradable material and stent design to develop larger diameter stents with reasonable profile and strength to sustain the vascular elastic forces.
- Long-term animal studies are warranted to confirm late positive remodeling and assess risks associated with stent fracture and stent fragment embolization during the degradation process.

INTRODUCTION

The advent of intravascular metal stents has revolutionized coronary interventions and pediatric and adult structural and congenital heart disease (CHD) interventions. Stents prevent immediate vessel recoil and provide better relief to obstruction when compared with balloon angioplasty alone, allowing for late positive remodeling. The disadvantages include early or late restenosis caused by neointimal hyperplasia, but most importantly, the permanent nature of these stents means late complications are always possible. A permanent metallic cage is an extreme limitation in a growing pediatric patient with CHD.

The quest for an ideal biodegradable stent (BDS) continues. The biggest theoretic advantage of BDS is that they disappear after their job is done. Thus, they initially provide mechanical support, broadly analogous to metallic stents in relieving vascular obstruction, but the long-term disadvantages of a fixed cage are avoided.

BDSs that are completely resorbed will also theoretically negate late complications: thrombosis,

Disclosure Statement: T.R. Welch, Founder of Tremedics Medical Devices company and owns the patent for the stent design. A.W. Nugent and S.R. Veeram Reddy have nothing to disclose.

[a] Department of Cardiovascular and Thoracic Surgery, University of Texas Southwestern Medical Center, 5323 Harry Hines Boulevard, Dallas, TX 75390, USA; [b] Division of Cardiology, Department of Pediatrics, Northwestern University Feinberg School of Medicine, Ann & Robert H. Lurie Children's Hospital of Chicago, 225 East Chicago Avenue, Box 21, Chicago, IL 60611, USA; [c] Division of Cardiology, Department of Pediatrics, University of Texas Southwestern Medical Center, Children's Health System of Texas, Childrens Medical Center, 1935 Medical District Drive, Dallas, TX 75235, USA
* Corresponding author.
E-mail address: SUREN.REDDY@CHILDRENS.COM

Intervent Cardiol Clin 8 (2019) 81–94
https://doi.org/10.1016/j.iccl.2018.08.009

bleeding problems associated with long-term anti-coagulation, permanently diminished flow of covered side branches,[1] permanent late fracture,[2] and computed tomography and MRI artifact. Furthermore, the lack of a metallic scaffold potentially allows for growth and normal vessel vasomotion.[3] Although spontaneous vessel growth after bioresorption may be possible, at the very least there will not be a fixed metallic cage that makes spontaneous growth impossible. Supportive evidence includes human coronary arteries with an enlarged lumen and normal vasomotion after 2 years, which suggest a healed endothelialized natural vessel[3] and porcine coronary arteries with positive remodeling after degradation and vessel growth.[4] The one certainty with resorption will be preservation of all future treatment options (unhindered surgery or additional interventions) because embedded metal stents create difficulties for surgeons and interventional cardiologists. Clearly, growing children with CHD have the most to gain from this technology.

Some of the known limitations of BDS include suboptimal mechanical characteristics with high recoil rate. To overcome recoil, thicker struts are used but these inherently pose problems with stent profile, stent delivery, increased local inflammation, which in turn cause restenosis, and reduced endothelial coverage.[5] Unfortunately for CHD applications, there are additional mechanical and engineering challenges to fabricate larger diameter BDSs that do not apply to small diameter BDSs. In addition, most of the polymer-based and magnesium-based BDSs are not radiopaque, which complicates accurate stent positioning in the catheterization laboratory and requires the addition of radiopaque markers.

CORONARY BIODEGRADABLE STENTS IN PEDIATRIC PATIENTS

Because of the potential to offer similar early outcomes and better late outcomes, BDSs have been studied extensively over past decades for coronary artery disease with only minimal reports in CHD. Case reports using coronary size bioresorbable (BR) stents off-label in Europe have emerged in very small infants with small vessels.[6–9] Multiple BDSs less than 4 mm diameter have undergone clinical trials[10–12] and are commercially available outside the United States. Zartner and colleagues[6,7] have described the use of the Biotronik stent, a magnesium corrodible stent made by Biotronik in Berlin, for stenting of a stenotic left pulmonary artery in a preterm infant as well as its pathology

several months after implantation. The same group also was the first to report the use of the same Biotronik stent for the treatment of an infant with recoarctation.[8] Despite these encouraging case reports, magnesium stents lose their structural integrity in several months and can cause a local tissue reaction as they degrade. Magnesium stents are also very difficult to visualize by fluoroscopy. The Biotronik stent was discontinued by Biotronik because of disappointing long-term results for the treatment of coronary disease but has now been replaced by a poly-L-lactic acid (PLLA)-coated, drug-eluting magnesium stent called Magmaris stent.

The Bioresorbable Vascular Scaffold (BVS) System (Abbott Vascular, Santa Clara, CA, USA) has undergone large trials in coronary arteries in randomized comparisons with cobalt-chromium everolimus-eluting stents.[10,11] The BVS has been commercially available outside the United States and obtained Food and Drug Administration (FDA) approval in July 2016. Although it was available, some congenital centers attempted to use the BVS for newborns with pulmonary arterial and venous disease. Although short-term stenting with BVS was successful in many instances, many of the lesions were found to have early restenosis with reports of stent migration.[9] In coronary artery disease, the BVS initially showed noninferiority but mounting evidence of increased early target lesion failure and late stent thrombosis[13] tempered enthusiasm and in September 2017 the company announced it will no longer be manufactured and distributed.

However, as shown in **Box 1**, there are ongoing bench testing, preclinical and clinical trials by many medical device companies across the globe to develop the ideal BDSs for coronary artery disease applications and much of this technology can be leveraged for pediatric stent technology.

Biodegradable/Bioresorbable Materials

Although the words biodegradable (BD) and bioresorbable (BR) provide similar meaning and are used interchangeably, they are technically different. A BD material is primarily degraded by a biological agent such as an enzyme or microbe. Bioresorption and bioabsorption is used to describe removal of degradation products by cellular activity, such as phagocytosis in a biological environment. A bioerodible or biocorrodible material is a water-insoluble substance that is converted in the body into a water-soluble material.[14] Different BD and BR

Box 1
Bioresorbable scaffolds in development, preclinical and clinical

- Igaki-Tamai, Kyoto Medical Planning Co., Kyoto, Japan
- BVS 1.1, Abbott Vascular, Santa Clara, CA USA
- Fortitude, Amaranth Medical, Mountain View, CA, USA
- Fantom Stent, Reva Medical, Inc., San Diego, CA, USA
- DeSolve Stent, Elixir Medical Corporation, Sunnyvale, CA, USA
- DREAMS 2G Stent, Biotronik AG, Bülach, Switzerland
- FAST Stent, Boston Scientific, Maple Grove, MN, USA
- MIRAGE Stent, Manli Cardiology Ltd, Singapore
- IBS Stent, Lifetech Scientific Co., Ltd, Shenzhen, China
- ART18Z Stent, Arterial Remodeling Technologies. Terumo, Tokyo, Japan
- Biolute, Biotronik, Bülach, Switzerland
- MeRes, Meril Life Science, Gujarat, India
- Arteriosorb, Arterius Limited, Leeds, London
- Ideal BioStent, Xenogenics Corp, Canton, MA, USA
- Xinsorb, Huaan Biotech, Upper Heyford, UK

See the following link to view images of these devices: https://www.sciencedirect.com/science/article/pii/S0167527316338049#f0020.

materials, primarily synthetic polymers or metals, have been tested and used for fabricating BDSs (Table 1).[15–22]

Synthetic polymers are mainly alpha hydroxy acids and the most commonly used polymer for fabricating stents is PLLA. Other polymers of particular interest for fabricating BD stents are polylactic acid (PLA), poly-D-lactic acid, polyglycolic acid (PGA), polyglycolic acid/polylactic acid, polydioxanone (PDS), polycaprolactone (PCL). The mechanical and thermal properties are important for the design of a BR stent. Materials such as PGA and PDS degrade rapidly over weeks to months, whereas others such as the PLA and PCL degrade over months to years. Controlling the degradation rate can aid in creating

Table 1
Mechanical and thermal properties for bioresorbable materials used for stents

Material	Young's Modulus (GPa)	Tensile Strength (MPa)	Melt Temperature (°C)	Glass Transition Temperature (°C)	Degradation Time (mo)	Elongation at Break (%)
PGA	6–7	90–110	225–230	35–40	4–6	1–2
PLLA	2.8–7	55–354	170–179	60–65	24–36	3.3–49
PDLA	1.4–2.8	25–40	50–60	50–60	12–16	2–6
50:50 PLGA	1.4–2.8	40–55	Amorphous	45–50	1–2	1–4
65:35 PLGA	1.4–2.8	40–55	Amorphous	45–50	3–4	–
75:25 PLGA	1.4–2.8	40–55	Amorphous	50–55	4–5	–
85:15 PLGA	1.4–2.8	40–55	Amorphous	50–55	5–6	2–6
PCL	0.2–0.4	25–35	58–63	−65 to −60	<24	>300%
PLLA-P4HB	1	36	Amorphous	34	<12	–
Iron	150–170	210	1535	–	>12	40
WE43 (Mg alloy)	40–50	220–230	–	–	~12	2–20
Pure Zn (Extruded)	104	120	419	–	–	60

acid by-products around the implant site, thus leading to a lower neointimal hyperplasia response. The use of BR materials for stents follows different resorption phases that theoretically lead ultimately to restoration of the normal vessel.

Lincoff and colleagues[15] have shown that the use of PLLA was safe and effective for use in porcine models and the use of PLLA has expanded from animal models to humans, being one of the most studied polymers for stents. PLLA is a semicrystalline polymer with amorphous and crystalline regions (Fig. 1). With the amorphous chains connecting the crystalline regions of the polymer providing structural strength. It has a high glass transition temperature (Tg) meaning at body temperature there is slow degradation (polymer degradation is much faster at temperatures higher than the Tg and slower when lower than the Tg). Another important parameter for degradation is the molecular weight (Mn),[16–19] because the average Mn directly relates to the chain scissioning of the polymer.[16–20]

After stent implantation, hydrolytic degradation, where water is absorbed into the polymer structure, is the first-stage attack on the ester linkages in the amorphous regions. The PLLA chain has hydrophilic end groups of carboxylic acid that are in the amorphous phase. This depolymerization via hydrolysis is noted by onset of further mass loss. When the fibers no longer have cohesive strength, chain scissioning starts to fragment PLLA into low-Mn sections. The next stage is the onset of mass loss and the attack of the crystalline regions. Once PLLA is broken into smaller chains, phagocytes can assimilate small particles to soluble monomeric anions. This soluble L-lactate is changed to pyruvate that enters the Krebs cycle and it eventually converted to carbon dioxide and water.

The resorption phase of PLLA is important because it controls the degradation rate. The slow degradation rate should prevent the buildup of degradation products that can lead to tissue damage or inflammation. During the degradation process the accelerated molecular weight loss leads to a reduction in radial strength overtime usually over 12 months shown in Fig. 2. The mass loss of the polymer is an indicator of the resorption process[21–26] and is a tradeoff for stents from a design and material perspective. Ideally, vessel patency remains while cellular tissue covers the stent and only then resorbs the material.

When developing larger diameter stents for pediatrics there are many design issues: large BRS have low radial strength, thus requiring thicker struts leading to difficulty in stent crimping/delivery and heightened inflammation; there are a lack of animal models of CHD for BRS testing; there are no safety studies for BRS embolization; and there is a possible need for antiproliferative drug-elution coating.

The most commonly used biocorrodible metals for BDS applications are magnesium, iron, and zinc.[27] The first metallic BDS implanted in humans was the absorbable magnesium coronary stent (AMS, Biotronik, Germany)[28] and as

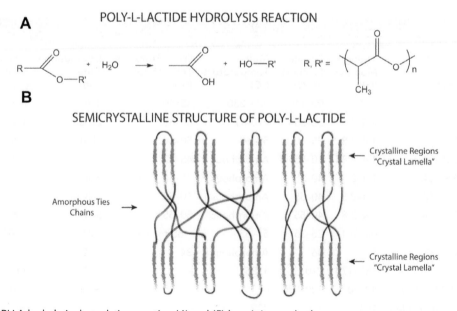

Fig. 1. PLLA hydrolysis degradation reaction (A) and (B) how it is resorbed.

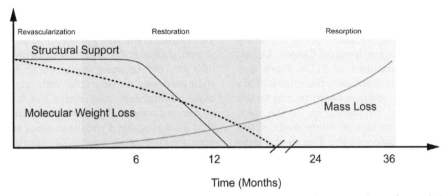

Fig. 2. Revascularization to resorption for bioresorbable stents during hydrolytic degradation for an aliphatic polyester, that is, PLLA.

previously discussed, was used off-label to treat pulmonary artery stenosis[6,7] and coarctation of aorta[8] with significant in-stent restenosis noted a few weeks later needing additional interventions. Other corrodible metals such as iron[29] and zinc[30,31] have shown some initial promise in animal preclinical testing. Different magnesium and zinc alloys continue to be tested in order to produce the ideal platform for use in a BDS. Metals can be alloyed with one another, coated with polymer and even manufactured with nanoparticles in order to optimize their strength, corrosion rates, radiopacity and ductility.

Limitations of Polymer-Based Biodegradable Stents

Polymer-based BDSs have limitations: lower radial strength with elastic recoil; unable to be viewed under fluoroscopic imaging; and limits to over dilation.[3] The Igaki-Tamai PLLA stent (Kyoto Medical Planning Co., Ltd., Kyoto, Japan), the first BRS implanted in human coronary arteries,[32] required increased strut thickness from 170 μm to 240 μm for sizes 5–8 mm diameter.[33] As these stents need heat to expand, their use has been limited. Also, PLLA stents manufactured with CO_2 laser cutting of a polymeric cylindrical shell, the method of choice for metal stents, melt the strut edges with nonuniform edges and crack formation risks strut failure.[34] New innovations in additive manufacturing and compression molding for stent designs have added interest for rapid manufacturing of stents. Most of the PLLA-based stents for 3 mm diameter are 150- to 180-μm thick that increases the profile and difficulty with delivery. Another limitation is that the expansion window of these stents is narrow. As stated earlier, metal stents implanted into pediatric patients are routinely overdilated.

Overexpansion of PLLA stents on implantation would cause stent fractures.[35] Therefore, appropriate vessel sizing initially is critical for BDSs.

Stents for Pediatric Applications

Infants and children born with CHD need larger diameter stents to dilate obstructed blood vessels such as the aorta and pulmonary arteries. There are many reasons that we continue to be without BDS scaffolds for pediatric applications. There are significant biomedical and engineering challenges related to decreasing collapse pressure and increasing elastic recoil with fabrication of larger diameter stents especially when constructed from polymers. As ideal absorption time is unknown, there are ongoing concerns for morbidity related to thromboembolism of the BDS fragments to distal vasculature and local reactions to the degrading stents. Furthermore, medical device companies continue to have reluctance to invest time and resources in a significantly small market size and the growing concern of the adult coronary artery BDS experience. However, there is a huge unmet need for a BDS in children and the bar is set very low because there currently is not a stent that we must compare with in order to show noninferiority.

Congenital pediatric interventionalists routinely use adult metallic coronary stents off-label in small pediatric patients and at follow-up deliberately fracture the cells with very high pressure balloons.[36–38] This deliberate breaking of metal stents with resultant sharp edges and risks of high-pressure dilations is merely a way to circumvent the unmet need that would be occupied by BDSs. Described below is a review of some of the work from different groups across the world who have been working toward fabricating a BDS for pediatric patients with CHD.

Tremedics Medical Devices

Illusicor (double opposed helical, DH) is a stent evaluated for CHD applications at the University of Texas Southwestern Medical Center, Dallas. The DH stent composed of PLLA fibers is a balloon expandable stent with the internal coils unfurling and expanding outward to add to the overall diameter of the stent (Fig. 3). The stent has platinum tip markers at either ends of the stents for fluoroscopic visibility. This stent design has overcome fabrication challenges posed to engineers to fabricate larger diameter stents for use in CHD. Engineering and preclinical analysis of this stent was initially in sizes from 3 to 8 mm diameter.[39–45] With a strut thickness of 100 μm, the collapse resistance at 3 to 4 mm diameter was comparable with commercially available stainless steel stents but less so at 5 to 6 mm diameter. There has been confirmation that increasing strut thickness leads to stronger stents with 8-mm diameter DH stents manufactured with strut thickness of 120 μm and

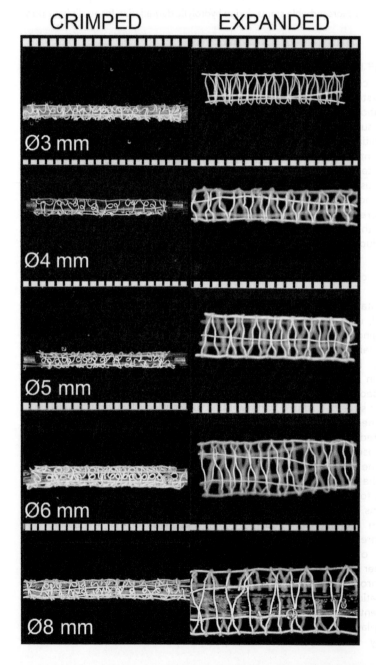

CRIMPED   **EXPANDED**

Ø3 mm

Ø4 mm

Ø5 mm

Ø6 mm

Ø8 mm

Fig. 3. The crimped and expanded DH stent sizes from 3–8 mm diameter made with 100 μm fiber. (*Courtesy of* Tremedics Medical Devices, North Richland Hills, TX; and *Adapted from* Welch T, Eberhart RC, Veeram Reddy SR, et al. Novel bioresorbable stent design and fabrication: congenital heart disease applications. Cardiovasc Eng Technol 2013;(4):174; with permission.)

Table 2
Mechanical properties of Illusicor (data reported at mean ± SD)

	Ø3 mm	Ø4 mm	Ø5 mm	Ø6 mm	Ø8 mm
Elastic Recoil (%)	0.48 ± 0.07	0.46 ± 0.1	1.6 ± 0.08	1.43 ± 0.14	3.0
Hoop Strength (ATM)	1.07 ± 0.02	0.80 ± 0.01	0.72 ± 0.02	0.63 ± 0.02	0.2

180 μm with improved recoil and collapse pressure[40] (Table 2). However, the challenge in pediatrics is to make these stents larger up to 20 mm diameter range.[46]

The single balloon-expandable DH stents show a decrease in collapse strength from 1.07 ± 0.02 (ATM) to 0.2 (ATM) for the 3- to 8-mm diameter DH stents at a strut thickness of 100 μm.[39,43] As stated earlier, the increase in the 8 mm strut to 180 μm showed an increase is collapse resistance to 0.75 ± 0.07 (ATM).[39] These data show that increasing the stent sizing with inner coils and strut thickness can maintain the hoop strength of the stent. Also increasing stent diameter and strut thickness leads to stronger stents and improved recoil.[39,40] The stent elastic recoil increased from 0.48% to 1.40% from 3 mm to 8 mm diameter. Overall target diameters were achieved with all stent sizes. The stents are composed of varying number of coils that unfurl during stent expansion (Fig. 4). This is an inherent feature of the stent design that permits this type of lengthening from 3.7% to 5% (see Fig. 4B).

To design a BR stent to meet the criterion for larger vessels, a larger strut thickness of 250 μm was examined. The rationale was based on the use of 240 μm strut thickness for the Genesis biliary stent for sizes 6 to 10 mm diameter. Fabricating thicker struts leads to increased absorption times, and although the ideal stent absorption time is unknown, there are some data to suggest that maintenance of structural integrity and strength for at least 6 months is desirable[3,44,47] and thus a reasonable goal. The required collapse pressure for clinical efficacy in CHD is also unknown but is likely significantly less than metal stents. Larger DH stents were fabricated to 10 and 14 mm diameter. The initial hoop strength was measured on an Instron RX 550/650 mechanical chamber analyzed with Blue Hill 3 software (Instron, Houston, TX) radial stent compression station. These stents are still under examination showing promising data as radial strength is maintained from 10 to 14 mm diameter with 0.32 ± 0.02 (N/mm) to 0.34 ± 0.02 (N/mm). Using the 250 μm and 300 μm struts there was no significant difference in radial strength for 10, 12, and 14 mm DH BRS.[48] Thus, the expected reduction in strength at larger diameters is somewhat controlled by the coil design.

Finite element analysis simulation
Another issue with BR stent design is the lack of structural simulation for these sizes. Finite Element Analysis (FEA) will allow better understanding of the stent interactions with an arterial wall. DH stent simulation was performed in Abaqus (Dassault Systemes Simulia Corp., Providence, RI, USA) and expanded to 3 mm diameter. Structural analysis of the DH stent

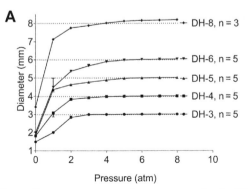
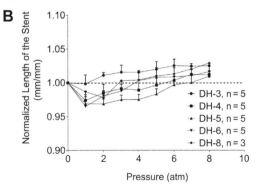

Fig. 4. The pressure versus diameter curves for the Ø3 to 8-mm DH stents (A) and normalized stent lengthening (B) DH stents expanded with a single-balloon catheter (data reported as mean ± SD). (*Adapted from* Welch T, Eberhart RC, Veeram Reddy SR, et al. Novel bioresorbable stent design and fabrication: congenital heart disease applications. Cardiovasc Eng Technol 2013;(4):176; with permission.)

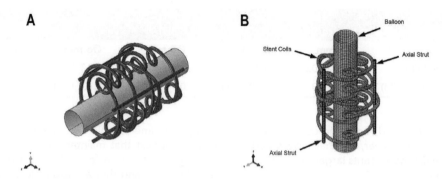

Fig. 5. The 3-dimensional solid model of the DH stent and a rigid surface for a balloon (*A*) and a finite element model showing the struts and stent coils (*B*).

was performed to better understand the interactions with an arterial wall and to show where the location of maximum hoop and von Mises stresses are in the model for potential areas of failure in the arterial layers as a result of this stent design. The DH stent was expanded with a balloon in the simulation (**Fig. 5**) and the artery was divided into 3 layers to represent the intima, media, and adventitia (**Figs. 6** and **7**).[47–50] The stent was expanded to a 3 mm diameter similar to previous animal testing in iliac arterial vessels. The simulation results showed the maximum stresses within the arterial walls was lower than the ultimate tensile strength. The intima layer experienced the highest hoop stress 247 kPa (**Fig. 8**) and von Mises stress of 276 kPa (**Fig. 9**), which is expected because it is in direct contact with the stent. The simulation results show similar deformation of the vessel comparable with the histologic results.[40] The preservation of the internal elastic lamina was shown in

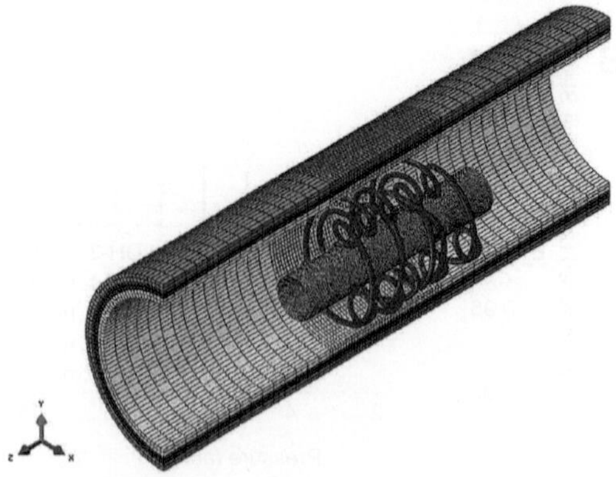

histologic results (**Fig. 10**) and thus expecting to yield a lower inflammation response.

Degraded stent's radial strength. PLLA stents have been bench tested for degradation showing a mass loss over 2 years (**Fig. 11**). The expected mass loss of the stents with 90 to 110 µm strut thickness is 3 to 3.5 years. Hydrolysis is the principal degradation mechanism for polyester such as PCL, PHB, and PLLA. Drawing PLLA fibers to smaller diameters creates a more crystalline-oriented structure that resists water penetration. This causes a slower degradation of these stents. Preliminary data on larger 10-mm diameter DH stents at 250 µm struts has shown an increase in hoop strength at 6 months and equivalent hoop strength at 1 year. The trend of increasing strength is likely the result from hydrolytic embrittlement of the stent during degradation.[51,52] This has been noticed by other experts in analyzing PLLA throughout degradation. Most other PLLA-based stents start losing structural integrity at 6 months,[10] but the Illusicor stent seems to maintain structural integrity at 1 year.

The Illusicor stent's increase in strength may also be due to the opposing coil design and use of fibers with a circular cross-sectional face instead of a laser cut PLLA tube with a rectangular cross-sectional face.

In-vivo preclinical testing. Preclinical tests on the above mentioned DH have been performed in iliac vessels, aorta, and lower descending aorta (LDA).[39,40,43,53] In-vivo testing shows the stent being deployable into rabbit and porcine models, being visible by use of radiopaque markers near the ends of the stent and resulting in good wall apposition by intravascular ultrasound (IVUS). There has been no significant

Fig. 6. The artery with 3 layers intima, media (red), and adventitia (green). The DH stent with the rigid balloon is shown with a high-density mesh within the area of contact with the artery.

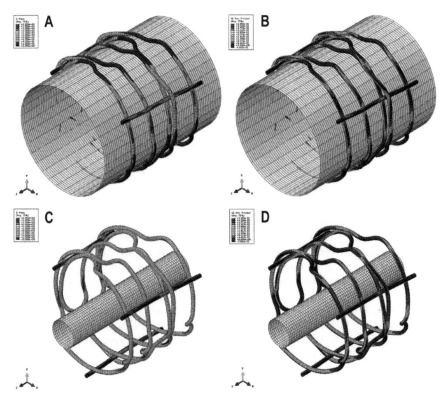

Fig. 7. The expanded stent von Mises stresses shown in (A) with plastically deformed regions shown in red with a maximum stress of 282 MPa and the total strain for the stent (B) showing the regional locations for PLLA plasticity in red. The maximum strain is 0.32. The relaxation analysis (C and D) shows the maximum von Mises stress is reduced to 195 MPa and the maximum strain remains at 0.32.

restenosis, stenosis or aneurysm, and resistance to downstream embolization.[39–41] The histologic results show mild inflammation of PLLA to surrounding tissue and as the stent structure degrades. DH stents of 8 mm diameter were implanted in porcine LDA, showing patent stents with no thrombosis and mild neointimal proliferation at 1 week, 1 month, and moderate neointimal proliferation at 9 months.[39] Coarctation of the aorta testing in minipig growth models was performed with 10-mm diameter metal Palmaz Genesis and DH stents implanted. At 1 year IVUS data showed that the Illusicor stent grows with the vessel and as expected, the metal stent does not grow with the vessel.[54,55] American Heart Association BGIA - The Lawrence J. and Florence A. De George Award 2015–2016. These results with the Illusicor stent are encouraging with regard to apposition, thrombosis, inflammation, and vessel growth. The Illusicor stent remains with structural integrity at 1 year with mild inflammation. These results with the

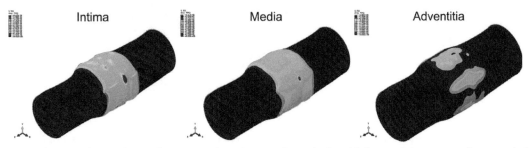

Fig. 8. The arterial circumferential stresses in the intima, media, and adventitia layers of the artery at the expanded state of the stent. The intima layer experiences the highest circumferential stresses. These stresses are reduced in the media and adventitia layers.

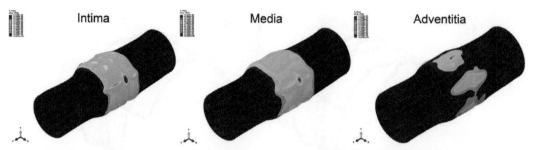

Fig. 9. The arterial von Mises stresses in the intima, media, and adventitia layers of the artery at the expanded state of the stent. The intima layer experiences the highest circumferential stresses. These stresses are reduced in the media and adventitia layers.

Illusicor stent are encouraging with regard to apposition, thrombosis, inflammation, and vessel growth. To design a BR stent to meet the criterion for larger vessels, a larger strut thickness of 300 μm are currently being evaluated for 10 to 20 mm diameter stent sizes.[47]

480 Biomedical (MA, USA)

With grant funding via the NHLBI SBIR pathway, the 480 Biomedical, Inc. (MA, USA) has developed and analyzed a pediatric resorbable scaffold (PRS, Fig. 12). This is a PLLA-based self-expanding stent with a unique composite design made of a PLLA fiber braid with elastomer coating that makes the stent as strong as the conventional metal stents used in pediatric practice but dissolves in 12 to 18 months. The stent is a composite consisting of braided fiber monofilaments of poly (L-lactide-co-glycolide) L-PLGA coated with poly (glycolide-co-caprolactone) PGCL.[56] The L-PLGA stents without a coating showed a chronic outward radial force of 90 mm Hg and a radial stiffness of 28 mm Hg. This improved to a radial stiffness of 700 mm Hg with a coating. The stent has radiopaque markers attached to the stent for visualization. The PRS stents were evaluated in native

pulmonary arteries in growing pigs showing excellent patency to 18-month full resorption with low inflammation score. The stents are currently being evaluated in animals to treat peripheral artery stenosis and coarctation and midterm results are expected this year. The stent is deliverable through a 5- or 6-Fr delivery system with an expanded diameter range of 7 to 10 mm and a length of 15 to 20 mm. The 480 Biomedical team reports that they are communicating with the FDA to initiate early feasibility first-in-human study. They plan to treat 10 subjects with PA stenosis with a Ø7X15 mm PRS and evaluate procedural success, safety at 1 month and patency at 6 months. They have also received NIH SBIR grant funding for the development of a similar stent scaffold designed specifically for the treatment of coarctation of the aorta in neonates. The work done at 480 Medical has not been published but has been presented at multiple national meetings.[57]

Akesys/Elixir Medical (CA, USA)

For coronary artery applications, Elixir Medical (CA, USA) evaluated the DESolve stent which is a novolimus-eluting BR coronary scaffold made of a PLLA-based polymer with good short-term

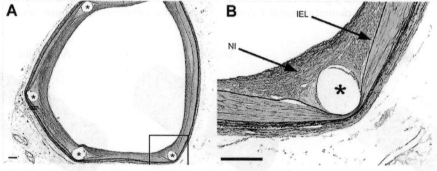

Fig. 10. Rabbit iliac artery sections show consistent stent-wall apposition. Hart's elastin stain (A) and (B) (magnified) show the neointimal response (NI) with an intact internal elastic lamina (IEL). Bar = 100 μm. (Adapted from Veeram Reddy SR, Welch TR, Wang J, et al. A novel biodegradable stent applicable for use in congenital heart disease: bench testing and feasibility results in a rabbit model. Catheter Cardiovasc Interv 2014;83(3):454; with permission.)

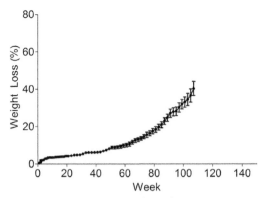

Fig. 11. Showing the weight loss of DH stents Ø3 mm, 100 μm fibers over 3 years (data reported as mean ± SD).

results. Akesys Medical with Elixir Medical subsequently developed a larger diameter (6 mm) stent, the balloon-expandable PRAVA Sirolimus Eluting Bioresorbable Peripheral Scaffold System that went into clinical trials in 2016 for treatment of superficial femoral artery disease. The company created a pediatric iteration, which was 5 to 6 mm diameter without drug, which was evaluated in porcine pulmonary arteries and abdominal aorta and demonstrated no

vessel inflammation and minimal vessel injury. By report (Kenny, personal communication, 2018) there is no further research planned, but there are plans for development of a pediatric iteration of the new hybrid design DynamX coronary stent, which uses polymer to hold joints of the stent together. In a similar fashion to the growth stent,[58] as the polymer is absorbed, the stent becomes flexible and fragmented.

Zinc Bioresorbable Stent/PediaStent

The newest biometal stent specifically designed for CHD is labeled the zinc BR stent or ZBS (Fig. 13). With NIH/SBIR funding, this stent is manufactured by PediaStent, a company formed in 2015, and made from a novel zinc alloy stent that harvests the natural antiinflammatory properties of zinc to attenuate neointimal hyperplasia response. Preliminary porcine study (Bocks, unpublished data, 2018) suggest that the ZBS has many attributes that would make it ideal for pediatric applications in CHD: higher radial strength, ultralow profile, radiopaque, low thrombogenicity, and minimal in-stent stenosis. Results of the PediaStent GLP animal study are eagerly awaited.

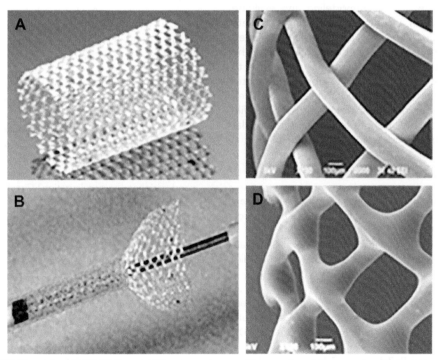

Fig. 12. 480 Biomedical PLGA/PLCL stent (A) mounted on a self-expanding delivery system (B). The scanning electron microscopy of the stent without coating (C) and with coating (D). (*Courtesy of* 480 Biomedical, Watertown, MA; and *Data from* Sharma U, Concagh D, Core L, et al. The development of bioresorbable composite polymeric implants with high mechanical strength. Nat Mater 2017;17:98; with permission.)

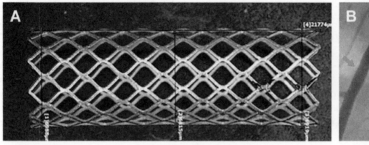

Fig. 13. Optical microscope picture of a 25 mm ZBS. (*A*) Following expansion on a 6 mm balloon. (*B*) Angiograms of iliac artery ZBS at 150 days postimplant (*orange arrow*). (*Courtesy of* [A] PediaStent, Cleveland, OH; and [B] Dr Martin Bocks, OH; with permission.)

SUMMARY

The quest for an ideal BDS for both adult coronary and pediatric CHD applications continues. Preclinical and clinical coronary studies showed late positive remodeling with normal vasomotor function after the stent disappears. BDSs are a very promising alternative to currently available metal stents to treat pediatric and adult patients with CHD, with the potential to eliminate the need for repeated interventions. Over the past few years, much progress has been made toward development of a dedicated pediatric BDS that can be used for CHD applications. Long-term animal studies are warranted to confirm late positive remodeling and evaluate vessel growth and function following complete stent degradation and assess risks associated with stent fragment embolization during the degradation process. Additional challenges to overcome include identifying optimal BD material (polymer vs metal) and stent design, developing larger diameter stents with low profile and reasonable strength to sustain the vascular elastic forces, and avoiding thrombosis.

REFERENCES

1. Law MA, Shamszad P, Nugent AW, et al. Pulmonary artery stents: long-term follow-up. Catheter Cardiovasc Interv 2010;75(5):757–64.

2. Breinholt JP, Nugent AW, Law MA, et al. Stent fractures in congenital heart disease. Catheter Cardiovasc Interv 2008;72(7):977–82.

3. Serruys PW, Ormiston JA, Onuma Y, et al. A bioabsorbable everolimus-eluting coronary stent system (ABSORB): 2-year outcomes and results from multiple imaging methods. Lancet 2009; 373(9667):897–910.

4. Strandberg E, Zeltinger J, Schulz DG, et al. Late positive remodeling and late lumen gain contribute to vascular restoration by a non-drug eluting bioresorbable scaffold: a four-year intravascular ultrasound study in normal porcine coronary arteries. Circ Cardiovasc Interv 2012;5(1):39–46.

5. Simon C, Palmaz JC, Sprague EA. Influence of topography on endothelialization of stents: clues for new designs. J Long Term Eff Med Implants 2000;10(1–2):143–51.

6. Zartner P, Cesnjevar R, Singer H, et al. First successful implantation of a biodegradable metal stent into the left pulmonary artery of a preterm baby. Catheter Cardiovasc Interv 2005;66(4):590–4.

7. Zartner P, Buettner M, Singer H, et al. First biodegradable metal stent in a child with congenital heart disease: evaluation of macro and histopathology. Catheter Cardiovasc Interv 2007;69(3): 443–6.

8. Schranz D, Zartner P, Michel-Behnke I, et al. Bioabsorbable metal stents for percutaneous treatment of critical recoarctation of the aorta in a newborn. Catheter Cardiovasc Interv 2006;67(5): 671–3.

9. McMahon CJ, Oslizlok P, Walsh KP. Early restenosis following biodegradable stent implantation in an aortopulmonary collateral of a patient with pulmonary atresia and hypoplastic pulmonary arteries. Catheter Cardiovasc Interv 2007;69(5):735–8.

10. Onuma Y, Serruys PW. Bioresorbable scaffold: the advent of a new era in percutaneous coronary and peripheral revascularization? Circulation 2011; 123(7):779–97.

11. Serruys PW, Onuma Y, Dudek D, et al. Evaluation of the second generation of a bioresorbable everolimus-eluting vascular scaffold for the treatment of de novo coronary artery stenosis: 12-month clinical and imaging outcomes. J Am Coll Cardiol 2011;58(15):1578–88.

12. Haude M, Erbel R, Erne P, et al. Safety and performance of the drug-eluting absorbable metal scaffold (DREAMS) in patients with de-novo coronary lesions: 12 month results of the prospective, multicentre, first-in-man BIOSOLVE-I trial. Lancet 2013; 381(9869):836–44.

13. Ali ZA, Serruys PW, Kimura T, et al. Two-year outcomes with the absorb bioresorbable scaffold for

treatment of coronary artery disease: a systematic review and meta-analysis of seven randomized trials with an individual patient data substudy. Lancet 2017;390:760–72.

14. Treiser M, Abramson S, Langer R, et al. Chapter I.2.6 - degradable and resorbable biomaterials A2 - Ratner, Buddy D. In: Hoffman AS, Schoen FJ, Lemons JE, editors. Biomaterials science. 3rd edition. London: Academic Press; 2013. p. 179–95.

15. Lincoff AM, Furst JG, Ellis SG, et al. Sustained local delivery of dexamethasone by a novel intravascular eluting stent to prevent restenosis in the porcine coronary injury model. J Am Coll Cardiol 1997; 29(4):808–16.

16. Weir NA, Buchanan FJ, Orr JF, et al. Degradation of poly-L-lactide. Part 2: increased temperature accelerated degradation. Proc Inst Mech Eng H 2004;218(5):321–30.

17. Weir NA, Buchanan FJ, Orr JF, et al. Degradation of poly-L-lactide. Part 1: in vitro and in vivo physiological temperature degradation. Proc Inst Mech Eng H 2004;218(5):307–19.

18. Weir NA, Buchanan FJ, Orr JF, et al. Processing, annealing and sterilisation of poly-L-lactide. Biomaterials 2004;25(18):39–49.

19. Tsuji H, Echizen Y, Nishimura Y. Photodegradation of biodegradable polyesters: a comprehensive study on poly(l-lactide) and poly(ε-caprolactone). Polym Degrad Stab 2006;91(5):1128–37.

20. Pitt CG, Zhong-wei G. Modification of the rates of chain cleavage of poly(ε-caprolactone) and related polyesters in the solid state. J Control Release 1987;4(4):283–92.

21. Garg S, Serruys PW. Coronary stents: current status. J Am Coll Cardiol 2010;56(10, Supplement):S1–42.

22. Hu T, Yang C, Lin S, et al. Biodegradable stents for coronary artery disease treatment: recent advances and future perspectives. Mater Sci Eng C Mater Biol Appl 2018;91:163–78.

23. Kenny D, Hijazi ZM. Bioresorbable stents for pediatric practice: where are we now? Interventional Cardiology 2015;7(3):245–55.

24. Naseem R, Zhao L, Liu Y, et al. Experimental and computational studies of poly-L-lactic acid for cardiovascular applications: recent progress. Mech Adv Mater Mod Process 2017;3(1):13.

25. Oberhauser JP, Hossainy S, Rapoza RJ. Design principles and performance of bioresorbable polymeric vascular scaffolds. EuroIntervention 2009; 5(Suppl F):F15–22.

26. Tsuji T, Tamai H, Igaki K, et al. Four-year follow-up of the biodegradable stent (Igaki-Tamai stent). Circ J 2004;68:135.

27. Bowen PK, Shearier ER, Zhao S, et al. Biodegradable metals for cardiovascular stents: from clinical concerns to recent Zn-alloys. Adv Healthc Mater 2016;5(10):1121–40.

28. Erbel R, Di Mario C, Bartunek J, et al. PROGRESS-AMS (Clinical performance and angiographic results of coronary stenting with absorbable metal stents) investigators. temporary scaffolding of coronary arteries with bioabsorbable magnesium stents: a prospective, non-randomised multicentre trial. Lancet 2007;369(9576):1869–75.

29. Peuster M, Hesse C, Schloo T, et al. Long-term biocompatibility of a corrodible peripheral iron stent in the porcine descending aorta. Biomaterials 2006;27(28):4955–62.

30. Bowen PK, Drelich J, Goldman J. Zinc exhibits ideal physiological corrosion behavior for bioabsorbable stents. Adv Mater 2013;25(18):2577–82.

31. Bowen PK, Guillory RJ 2nd, Shearier ER, et al. Metallic zinc exhibits optimal biocompatibility for bioabsorbable endovascular stents. Mater Sci Eng C Mater Biol Appl 2015;56:467–72.

32. Nishio S, Kosuga K, Igaki K, et al. Long-term (>10 years) clinical outcomes of first-in-human biodegradable poly-l-lactic acid coronary stents: igaki-tamai stents. Circulation 2012;125(19):2343–53.

33. Biamino G, Schmidt A, Scheinert D. Abstracts: international congress XVIII on endovascular interventions. J Endovasc Ther 2005;12(Supplement I): I1–50.

34. Grabow N, Schlun M, Sternberg K, et al. Mechanical properties of laser cut poly(L-lactide) microspecimens: implications for stent design, manufacture, and sterilization. J Biomech Eng 2005;127(1): 25–31.

35. Moore SS, O'Sullivan KJ, Verdecchia F. Shrinking the supply chain for implantable coronary stent devices. Ann Biomed Eng 2016;44(2):497–507.

36. Sathanandam SK, Haddad LM, Subramanian S, et al. Unzipping of small diameter stents: an in vitro study. Catheter Cardiovasc Interv 2015; 85(2):249–58.

37. Danon S, Gray RG, Crystal MA, et al. Expansion characteristics of stents used in congenital heart disease: serial dilation offers improved expansion potential compared to direct dilation: results from a pediatric interventional cardiology early career society (PICES) investigation. Congenit Heart Dis 2016;11(6):741–50.

38. Morray BH, McElhinney DB, Marshall AC, et al. Intentional fracture of maximally dilated balloon-expandable pulmonary artery stents using ultra-high-pressure balloon angioplasty: a preliminary analysis. Circ Cardiovasc Interv 2016;9(4):e003281.

39. Herbert CE, Reddy SV, Welch TR, et al. Bench and initial preclinical results of a novel 8 mm diameter double opposed helical biodegradable stent. Catheter Cardiovasc Interv 2016;88(6):902–11.

40. Veeram Reddy SR, Welch TR, Wang J, et al. A novel biodegradable stent applicable for use in congenital heart disease: bench testing and feasibility

results in a rabbit model. Catheter Cardiovasc Interv 2014;83:448–56.

41. Veeram Reddy SR, Welch TR, Wang J, et al. A novel design biodegradable stent for use in congenital heart disease: mid-term results in rabbit descending aorta. Catheter Cardiovasc Interv 2015;85:629–39.

42. Welch T, Eberhart R, Reisch J, et al. Influence of thermal annealing on the mechanical properties of PLLA coiled stents. Cardiovasc Eng Technol 2014;5(3):270–80.

43. Welch T, Eberhart RC, Veeram Reddy SR, et al. Novel bioresorbable stent design and fabrication: congenital heart disease applications. Cardiovasc Eng Technol 2013;(4):171–82.

44. Welch T, Eberhart RC, Chuong CJ. Characterizing the expansive deformation of a bioresorbable polymer fiber stent. Ann Biomed Eng 2008;36(5):742–51.

45. Welch TR, Eberhart RC, Chuong CJ. The influence of thermal treatment on the mechanical characteristics of a PLLA coiled stent. J Biomed Mater Res B Appl Biomater 2009;90(1):302–11.

46. Shibbani K, Kenny D, McElhinney D, et al. Identifying gaps in technology for congenital interventions: analysis of a needs survey from congenital interventional cardiologists. Pediatr Cardiol 2016;37(5):925–31.

47. Nugent AW, Welch T. Development of large diameter bioresorbable stents for congenital heart diease. J Am Coll Cardiol 2018;71(11 Supplement):A1353.

48. Gervaso F, Capelli C, Petrini L, et al. On the effects of different strategies in modelling balloon-expandable stenting by means of finite element method. J Biomech 2008;41(6):1206–12.

49. Holzapfel GA, Sommer G, Gasser CT, et al. Determination of layer-specific mechanical properties of human coronary arteries with nonatherosclerotic intimal thickening and related constitutive modeling. Am J Physiol Heart Circ Physiol 2005;289(5):H2048–58.

50. Welch TR, Eberhart RC, Banerjee S, et al. Mechanical interaction of an expanding coiled stent with a plaque-containing arterial wall: a finite element analysis. Cardiovasc Eng Technol 2016;7(1):58–68.

51. Pan P, Zhu B, Inoue Y. Enthalpy relaxation and embrittlement of poly(l-lactide) during physical aging. Macromolecules 2007;40(26):9664–71.

52. Pan H, Na B, Lv R, et al. Embrittlement of poly (L-lactide)/poly (ε-caprolactone) blends upon physical aging. J Polymer Res 2012;19(8):9936.

53. DeSena HC, Reddy SV, Welch T, et al. Inflammatory response of biodegradable stents in the ductus arteriosus in a neonatal piglet model. J Am Coll Cardiol 2013;61(10_S).

54. Veeram Reddy SR, Welch TR, Wang J, et al. Porcine model of aortic coarctation: treatment with novel biodegradable stent up to 12mm diameter. Circulation 2016;134:A18924.

55. Veeram Reddy SR, Welch T, Wang J, et al. Novel biodegradable stent for treatment of congenital heart disease – 1 year results in porcine model of coarctation of aorta. J Struct Heart Dis 2016;2(6):289.

56. Sharma U, Concagh D, Core L, et al. The development of bioresorbable composite polymeric implants with high mechanical strength. Nat Mater 2017;17:96.

57. Ratnayaka. Purpose-built bioresorbable elastomer-polymer stent for aortic coarctation and pulmonary artery stenosis. Chicago: PICS-AICS Symposium; 2014.

58. Ewert P, Riesenkampff E, Neuss M, et al. Novel growth stent for the permanent treatment of vessel stenosis in growing children: an experimental study. Catheter Cardiovasc Interv 2004;62(4):506–10.

Printed and bound by CPI Group (UK) Ltd, Croydon, CR0 4YY

03/10/2024

01040304-0015